DADS, KIDS, AND FITNESS

DADS, KIDS, AND FITNESS

A Father's Guide to Family Health

WILLIAM MARSIGLIO

R

RUTGERS UNIVERSITY PRESS

New Brunswick, New Jersey, and London

Library of Congress Cataloging-in-Publication Data
Names: Marsiglio, William, author.
Title: Dads, kids, and fitness : a father's guide to family health / William Marsiglio.
Description: New Brunswick, New Jersey : Rutgers University Press, [2016] | Includes
bibliographical references and index.
Identifiers: LCCN 2016003237| ISBN 9780813584867 (hardcover : alk. paper) | ISBN
9780813584874 (e-book (ePub)) | ISBN 9780813584881 (e-book (Web PDF))
Subjects: LCSH: Families—Health and hygiene. | Father and child. |
Physical fitness. | Health.
Classification: LCC RA777.7 .M37 2016 | DDC 613.7—dc23
LC record available at https://lccn.loc.gov/2016003237

A British Cataloging-in-Publication record for this book is available from the British
Library.

Visit our website: http://rutgerspress.rutgers.edu

Manufactured in the United States of America

To my mother, Marguerite Grace Marsiglio, who during her ninety-two years of life modeled a style of devoted parenting that taught me how to be a nurturing dad; and to my two sons, Scott Michael and Phoenix Jesse, who have inspired me to embrace a healthy lifestyle.

CONTENTS

PREFACE

My decision to write a book that explores the intersection of fathers' and children's health and fitness stems from my scholarly interests as well as my life as both a man and a father. Understanding how fathers think, feel, and act has been at the center of my research agenda. Looking at fathers' approaches to health in *Dads, Kids, and Fitness: A Father's Guide to Family Health* extends my most recent writing, in which I challenge fathers to move beyond their bread-winning role to become a more nurturing force for their children. On a personal front, I reveal in my current work my passion for the sports and fitness worlds as a participant, fan, and over the last six years, a youth coach. Ever since my boyhood days, I've committed myself to being healthy and fit.

Inspired by this mix of professional and personal sentiments, I began to envision my project a number of years ago. In February 2008, I had a student assistant do a few pilot interviews with fathers that focused on their orientation toward their own health as well as their children's health. During the next several years, two other students conducted similar interviews with other dads for me. In all, I compiled stories from twelve fathers about health- and fitness-related matters.

The pilot interviews piqued my curiosity and convinced me that dads could share intimate and meaningful insights about critical issues that interest me. Unfortunately, it wasn't until March 2012 that I personally had a chance to interview a father about health and fitness topics. That interview confirmed for me that there was a big story to tell about how fathers and children in the United States can shape, for better or worse, each other's well-being by their approach to disability, eating, exercise, formal and informal health care, risk taking and safety practices, sleep patterns, and more. Over the next eighteen months, I interviewed a diverse sample of 102 dads and pediatric health care professionals across the country. I am grateful to a University of Florida semester sabbatical for giving me the flexibility to complete all the interviews myself in a timely way. I finished my last interview in September 2013.

Beginning with my pilot research and continuing throughout all the writing stages, I was fortunate to receive excellent help from twenty-seven undergraduate and graduate students. Once I started talking to dads, I challenged my team of assistants to choose a moniker for themselves to enhance our espirit de corps. They enthusiastically morphed into the Avengers, expressing their intense dedication to the project, a sentiment that subsequent cohorts of Avengers replicated. The Avengers helped with recruitment, transcription, data management, literature searches, conceptual development, manuscript review and editing, and other tasks. As young adults, some sharpened my sensitivity to various concerns relevant to dads and kids. They sometimes also challenged me to alter the style and substance of my narrative. In multiple ways, the Avengers were a vital asset. Indeed, without the Avengers' assistance, the project might not have been possible, and its quality certainly less. I'm deeply grateful for their diligent efforts, ideas, inspiration, and emotional support. I extend a heartfelt thanks to Kayti Agnelli, Ethan Blauner, Jessie Carnevale, Chris Errico, Carolina De La Rosa, Karine DeSouza, William French, Lauren Gilbert, Justin Hendricks, Medjine Jarbath, Annabeth Johnson, Deepika Kulkarni, Christine Latham, Luke Liberty, Caitlyn LoMonte, Mindy Maconi, Tilman Monsanto, Jesus Moises, Sam Morris, Daniel Perry, Matt Rafferty, Jacyln Ramos, Miranda Schonbrun, Erica Self, Mariann Strange, Haley Sterling, Brionca Taylor, Catherine "Cat" Walter, Leighton Williams, Seth Wood, and Tom Young. I also wish to thank Sheryl McIntosh, my department's former office manager, for her efficient and friendly contributions, which helped me manage various aspects of the Avengers' participation.

Two other people were instrumental in bringing this project to fruition. I'm grateful to Peter Mickulas, senior editor at Rutgers University Press, who expressed his enthusiasm for this project immediately and continued to assist me effectively as I navigated the production process. My copy editor, Willa Speiser, provided extensive, thoughtful, meticulous, and candid editorial guidance that improved this book considerably. I appreciate her keen literary eye and how she gently forced me to rethink and rewrite my ideas while offering useful substantive suggestions of her own.

My goal is to encourage dads from diverse backgrounds to become more self-conscious about their health and fitness and to enhance their ability to monitor and support their children's well-being in these areas. When I hear dads describe their engaged or limited involvement with their kids, and when I listen to pediatric health care professionals' comments about dads, I become even more introspective about my own choices and experiences as a father. I trust that readers will also relate to and learn from the accounts I present.

Because I want to entice a broad audience to embrace the idea that dads should do more to promote their kids' health and fitness, I integrate snippets of my own life as a father of two sons into my larger message about the fathers' experiences I represent in the book. When readers consider my firsthand stories about how I've navigated being a father, I want them to see that my perspective is grounded in my professional expertise as well as my experiential sense of fathering. I also want readers to appreciate more fully the varied options and constraints fathers face in making a difference in their children's lives.

One of the unexpected benefits of writing this book was that in fall 2014 I launched my *Dads & Kids: Health & Fitness Talk* website (http://www .dadsandkidshealth.com/) and Facebook page (https://www.facebook .com/dadsandkidshealth). Starting in the winter of 2016, I could also be found @DadsKidsHealth on Twitter. The website, in my own words, is "an interactive web resource to inform and inspire individuals committed to promoting healthy lifestyles for fathers and children." After finishing the first draft of my manuscript, I started to blog about my experiences on the website and several of the initial blogs compelled me to refine the text in my final draft.

I wrote *Dads, Kids, and Fitness* and developed the Internet and social media resources with a similar purpose in mind—to bridge the divide between academic research and people's everyday lives so that fathers and children might adopt healthier perspectives and practices. By championing ideas and creating practical outlets, I want to foster a community of like-minded men and dads who will individually and collectively nurture a generation of healthier children. Dads need to be encouraged to become more introspective about their fathering, to talk to one another in a supportive spirit about their experiences, and to relate to their kids in new and productive ways about health and fitness.

DADS, KIDS, AND FITNESS

1 ❧ MAPPING DADS' PLACE IN THE HEALTH MATRIX

W̲HEN MY SECOND SON, Phoenix, was born in 2007, I became a forty-nine-year-old later-life dad. Phoenix's birth inspired me to reframe my outlook on fitness and healthy living; my one-hour, high-tempo rides on my blue Trek 1500 road bike were now a practical sign of "good fathering." Painting on sunscreen, wearing a helmet, and prioritizing safe roads for my rides had a meaning beyond my wife and me. I knew that whatever happened to me would also leave an imprint on my infant son.

In addition to meeting my responsibilities as a nurturing dad, I was determined to stay fit. No way, I thought, am I going to bank on good luck and good genes to ensure my active role in Phoenix's life journey. I reject being a feeble old man, or worse yet, dead, as Phoenix stamps his mark on the world.

My philosophy took root years ago. As an adolescent I witnessed my paternal grandfather, Nono, a veteran of World War I, succumb to a hard life of coal mining, excessive drinking, and sedentary leisure. He was left a broken, bitter man, dying at age eighty-two. His final years left me with cloudy memories of awkward visits to a dreary veterans' nursing home. Little dignity comes with wasting away in bed or shuffling corridors in a drab gown and slippers for over five years. The black lung, tuberculosis, and other ailments—some most likely self-inflicted—cut off all the energy that had previously lingered in his self-abused, middle-aged body. Perhaps his fate would have been different had my grandmother not unexpectedly preceded him in death by fifteen years. No doubt good genes and stubbornness kept him alive much longer than life expectancy charts would predict.

My dad, who witnessed Nono's destructive lifestyle and demise, came to see a manly life differently than I eventually did. An infantryman in World War II who fought in the Battle of the Bulge, Dad was part of what American television journalist Tom Brokaw termed the "Greatest Generation." After returning from the war, Dad survived four decades of sweaty days and nights doing manual labor at the General Tire & Rubber Company (referred to locally as the Rubber Works) in Jeannette, Pennsylvania. Built in the early 1900s, this hot, dingy factory wore down those who took their work seriously.

Dad, like many men of his era, embraced his position as the family's sole breadwinner. With few exceptions, he cashed in on opportunities to take overtime, double shifts, and weekend work. Many of those grueling days at the plant were "celebrated" by nights of heavy drinking in downtown bars.

An accomplished athlete in his youth, Dad's time playing sports competitively ended long before my birth. Regrettably, I never saw him truly exercise beyond playing catch with me. Hours of manual labor left him with no appetite for fitness training or active play. Nor do I recall him saying much of anything about healthy eating as it related to him, others, or me. He surely never lifted a hand to plan or prepare a meal, and I have absolutely no memory of Dad being a caregiver on the rare instances when I was either sick or injured.

When it came to sports, I was expected to self-motivate if I wanted to practice or play. To his credit, when he wasn't working, Dad attended my games and sometimes even helped coach my youth baseball teams. In keeping with the standards of the day, Dad positioned himself as the conventional husband and father who relegated domestic caretaking activities to Mom, who was a full-time homemaker. Fortunately, even though I have no childhood memories of him being my caregiver or showing me affection, I never doubted Dad's love.

My most vivid childhood memory of Dad's fitness involves my routinely asking him to "make a muscle." I harbor deep memories of the adulation I felt when my tiny hands grasped his rock-hard biceps. I longed to possess such power when I grew to be a man. As a child, I was unfazed that he didn't exercise for fun. He was the sturdy oak tree in my life, never sick or weak. In my gendered world, it never dawned on me that Mom might have been the one to show me a parental exercise model—though that possibility is moot because she never exercised either. There's no telling if I might have become an even bigger exercise junkie had my parents devoted themselves to health and fitness.

Fortunately, thanks to my doting mother and a generous pension with impressive health care benefits, Dad got what he needed to outlive his father by almost a decade. He also lived a healthier life, despite being overtaken by dementia and cancer in his later years. Yet as I moved into and beyond my young adult years, I saw that my father's approach to health and fitness, even if it was a step up from Nono's, left much to be desired. All told, I witnessed only a minor generational shift in how the older men in my life managed their bodies and health.

I was determined to pursue a different path. By choice and circumstance I avoided the stress of military service and the years of exhausting, blue-collar labor. I had my taste of roofing, construction, and landscaping jobs as a high school and college student and knew I wanted no part of that lifestyle in the long term. Fortunately, federal aid and loans made it possible for me to pursue my formal education. As a student and later an academic, my flexible schedule gave me untold opportunities to carve out time to engage in exercise as leisure, which I did.

For me, exercise is a daily ritual, a physical and mental fix despite my chronic problems with cramping calves and a vulnerable lower back. Unfortunately, my early thirties greeted me with physical ailments that forced me to curtail my athletic options and eventually complicated my life as a hands-on, sports-loving dad. I've had to forgo my long runs, serious pickup basketball games, and competitive tennis because I can no longer do those activities without subjecting myself to excruciating leg cramps and back pain. Although the alternatives are far from ideal, I've been able to remain physically active with Phoenix directly through cycling and swimming, and I've been a formal and informal coach for his basketball, flag football, soccer, tennis, and triathlon adventures.

THE FATHER-CHILD HEALTH MATRIX

With my own life as an example, this book is only partly about how men, or fathers in particular, perceive and manage their own health. It explores several other related and equally compelling questions: How do fathers perceive, attend to, and influence their daughters' and sons' health, fitness, and general sense of well-being? How are fathers' lifelong personal experiences of taking care of or abusing their own bodies and minds related to the way they take care of their children's health-related needs? How do fathers and mothers navigate the world of coparenting when dealing with their children's health? What can be done to enhance fathers' opportunities to forge a legacy that enriches how their children see and treat their bodies and minds?

These questions intrigue me because I am a social scientist who studies the social aspects of fathering. Yet these issues are also distinctly personal to me, both as a man and as a father. Every day I am reminded of my gains and losses as I strive to steady my fitness profile for as long as possible while Phoenix, my younger son, grows into his body and out of his clothes. With each step I lose in our race across the field, he gains one. My mission as a father, similar to what many fathers of young children say to me, is to help my son make healthy choices that will enrich his life for years to come.

Fulfilling that mission is no easy task, for me or others. Fathers, as men, face all sorts of competing pressures from family, friends, peers, coworkers, and social institutions that all too often weaken their ability to be effective caregivers and messengers of a healthy lifestyle. And we can't ignore the effect of money, or the lack thereof. Poor finances set in motion a nasty web of constraints that alter the kinds of choices fathers can make for themselves and their families. Many fathers struggle to obtain adequate health care, secure a safe living environment, and purchase fresh, healthy foods, which are usually more expensive than other food options. Sometimes those entrenched in the ranks of the working poor are trapped into juggling work schedules for two or three jobs. When can these exhausted, sleep-deprived fathers find time to exercise without ignoring their partners and kids?

Despite our wealth as a nation, far too many children as infants, toddlers, grade-schoolers, and adolescents experience poor outcomes in their emotional, mental, and physical health. Initially, this is seen in high rates of infant mortality and low birth-weight babies. The bad news continues for the alarmingly high rates of kids who are obese, get pregnant, contract a sexually transmitted disease, smoke, binge drink, abuse drugs, develop an eating disorder, or attempt suicide.[1]

Sadly, many of the adult men young people look to, including their fathers, are poor role models. They are ill-equipped to help kids avoid or correct unhealthy behaviors. However, as the stories I share in this book reveal, many fathers can, and do, lead by example. They can be caring, attentive, and inspirational beacons for their children's healthy lifestyle.

Kids have some control over a number of circumstances that influence the quality of their health, but many youth suffer from chronic illnesses not of their own doing. Their only real "choice" comes by way of the decisions they make to manage the effects of their condition. Estimates vary, but about one in every four or five kids in America lives with some type of chronic illness.[2] Some are "normalized" conditions like asthma and diabetes;[3] others, including cystic fibrosis and muscular dystrophy, tend to shorten a person's life.[4] Fathers in most of these situations, whether resident or nonresident, are likely to make a difference in their children's lives, for either better or worse. True, many fathers are missing in action when it comes to caring for chronically ill children, but in the past few years I've gained a newfound respect for the numerous fathers who have risen to the challenge of caring for children who have been stricken with paralysis, type 1 diabetes, cancer, Down syndrome, cerebral palsy, autism, and other troubling physical, mental, and emotional conditions. Some of these men even match the incredible care usually provided by mothers of children with severe disabilities.

My purpose in writing this book is to breathe new life into the complex debate about fathers, children, and health. To be clear, in my everyday life, and in this book, I often hold men accountable for their poor health habits while applauding the men who have committed themselves to nurturing their own and their children's health. I hope that all fathers, even those who work many hours for pay, will be involved in a healthy style of caregiving that benefits their children physically, emotionally, psychologically, and spiritually. As I see it, men can make choices that are likely to help their children live healthier lives. But men, some more than others, also face real constraints beyond their immediate control that limit their ability to bring about positive health outcomes for their children.

I purposely set out to sample an eclectic group of fathers to help me better understand what I've come to call the social health matrix. The

Merriam-Webster dictionary tells us that a matrix is "something within or from which something else originates, develops, or takes form." I explore that portion of the health matrix most clearly marked by the myriad conditions, relationships, and choices that define matters of health, fitness, and well-being for fathers' and children's intersecting lives.

Exploring the social matrix for health, fitness, and well-being issues is challenging because these topics are multilayered and fluid. In its constitution, the World Health Organization notes that "health is a state of complete physical, mental and social well-being and not merely the absence of disease or infirmity."[5] At first glance this sounds reasonable and straightforward, yet our complex world is marked by numerous competing and shifting images about what is healthy and unhealthy, fit and unfit. Is it really possible to "know" precisely what it means to be healthy or fit? Some, perhaps many, believe there is no definitive, objective standard for what constitutes good health or fitness. These are contested states of being, or perhaps continua of experience, that are affected by historical and cultural developments anchored to an assortment of values, knowledge, technology, and behavior. As Jonathan Metzl, a professor of sociology and medicine, astutely asserts, "health" is a "term replete with value judgments, hierarchies, and blind assumptions that speak as much about power and privilege as they do about well-being. Health is a desired state, but it is also a prescribed state and an ideological position."[6]

Meanings of health and fitness can also be seen as matters of personal preference that are often tied to moral assumptions about good and bad behavior. We often define our own health by portraying others' health as not up to a particular standard or spoiled in some way.[7] We might also interpret our own health status as falling below that of our friends, family, or some generic vision of others whom we hold in high regard.

Nonetheless, common sense tells us that people typically perceive forms of misery and pain—whether physical, emotional, or mental—as undesirable and that some level of contentment with one's physical, emotional, and mental states of being is consistent with good or at least acceptable health. Of course people differ in terms of the thresholds they need to feel "contentment" and pleasure, but almost everyone agrees that certain conditions or states of being are preferable to others. For example, it's preferable to be able to walk up a flight of stairs without feeling out of breath. It's preferable to have the mobility to complete everyday tasks without pain or assistance.

It's preferable to be emotionally and psychologically calm and confident with one's place in the world. It's preferable to wake up in the morning and look forward to the day optimistically. More generally, it's preferable to live a longer and healthier life than to be burdened by ailments and disabilities that curtail one's lifespan and quality of life. Being in good health and relatively content, irrespective of how people perceive these conditions, often means that people feel they have some degree of control over their minds and bodies and are experiencing some type of pleasure.

Viewing health and fitness as commodities in a capitalist context adds another dimension to how meaning is assigned to these states of being. Profit systems attached to health, nutrition, and fitness try to define what matters most and why. These profit systems are shaped by forces of social control that are tied to institutions within diverse sectors (media, medicine, fitness industry, and education) and the health care professionals, counselors, personal trainers, educators, and others who work for them. The personnel connected to these institutions are influential when they help establish norms and regulate conduct. Plenty of "experts," both credentialed and self-proclaimed, assert their opinions on diet, exercise, sleep, health care products, injuries, diseases, therapies, and more. They also affect what standards and forms of measurement are used and valued when assessing health quality and fitness levels.

Whatever particular standards are applied, some people will get labeled as being sick, having ADHD, being unfit and obese, eating poorly, or having some other undesirable physical or mental condition. Generally speaking, the labeling process unfolds differently for people based on their social standing and access to resources. Poor, less educated adults and children are more likely than their more affluent counterparts to be judged as or determined to be unhealthy.[8] Once people are identified as falling outside the norm, how are they persuaded or forced to conform to a range deemed "normal" for a particular condition? Social and marketing pressures abound to get "deviants" to address their negative circumstances so they can get healthier and fitter.

Although these types of broad social and institutional concerns shape the American landscape of health and fitness, I focus this book primarily on the family-based realities of how dads and kids think, talk, and act in the health matrix. I reveal much about fathers' and children's real-life experiences while encouraging dads to become more health and fitness conscious for themselves and their families. In the process, I highlight the cultural and social challenges some fathers face in achieving this pro-health orientation in an American context.

FOUR KEY PARTNERSHIPS

Because fathering is a social arrangement influenced by other people, institutions, and culture, I show how four types of partnerships (father-child, father-coparent, father–non-family members, and community organizations' interactions) affect fathers' and children's life experiences in the health matrix. Most importantly, a motivated father tries to create what essentially is a goal-oriented partnership with his child—even though he is unlikely to call it that. Ideally, the child will follow the father's lead and gradually embrace shared goals about matters like nutrition, exercise, sleep, and personal safety that they can cooperatively try to achieve. Primitive signs of this happening can be discerned once the child communicates and reasons like a typical four- or five-year-old. As the child matures, the prospects for a more reciprocal partnership will, too. In time the father may perceive himself as more of a resource for his increasingly independent child. This partnership, like the others a father can create with coparents and personnel working in community organizations, is most likely to flourish when each partner values what the other has to offer as they share responsibility and accountability for decision making.

Some men are decidedly more aware than others of what they want to accomplish as fathers. Those with a plan are better prepared and more eager to develop a partnership with their children. However, a partnership is a joint affair; a child's personality can dictate whether a cooperative spirit emerges. Some kids are much more likely than others to accept guidance from their fathers about health and fitness goals. The father who expresses little, if any, interest in his child's health and fitness is unlikely to establish a true partnership. Nonetheless, this type of father may negatively affect his child's health. The obese father is unlikely to encourage his child explicitly to follow in his footsteps, but his actions and comments might still reinforce his child to eat poorly and spend less time exercising.

Most dads, even many single dads, have some type of relationship with the mother of their child, another parental figure, or sometimes both. How fathers navigate their coparental partnerships can affect the messages children receive about diet, exercise, safety issues, and disease maintenance as well as the outcomes they experience. In today's age, such partnerships have become much more complicated because people increasingly move into and out of various family and household arrangements.

Good fathering extends beyond the family and household. Fathers have opportunities to nurture different types of partnerships with medical professionals, educators, coaches, youth ministers, and others who play a role in shaping children's approach to health, fitness, and well-being. In almost all families, if a father is truly interested in his child's well-being he can find a way to serve as his child's advocate to those in the community who can enhance the child's life.

Finally, dads can be targeted by agencies and organizations that partner with one another on behalf of children. For example, a partnership between a local school system and a public health department or food co-op could encourage a father (and mother) to join the child at school to help plant and maintain a garden. An engaged father might even take the initiative to create bridges between organizations that would expand opportunities for his child.

ABOUT THE RESEARCH

These pages are filled with stories of joy, sadness, courage, irresponsibility, and perseverance that are intimately tied to the health matrix. To offer a full account of how fathers' health matters to them and their kids, I incorporate the words of healthy fathers as well as the tales of dads who struggle with chronic illnesses and physical impairments. Similarly, I consider how fathers relate to their healthy children in addition to telling the stories of fathers whose children have chronic illnesses like autism, cancer, cerebral palsy, and diabetes or manage severe conditions such as paralysis, blindness, deafness, and obesity. Although I accentuate the social and psychological transformation of boys into men who become fathers, I explore fathers' experiences raising daughters as well as sons.[9]

The stories I present come from fathers who range in age from twenty-two to sixty. These fathers differ widely in their level of formal schooling, the types of places where they grew up and currently live, their family composition and financial status, race and ethnic heritage, religious views, and sexual orientations. I spoke with doctors, managers, computer experts, stock clerks, business consultants, mechanics, personal trainers, the unemployed, and more. Some have teenage and young adult children; others push youngsters in strollers. One father, basking in the afterglow of becoming a dad, spoke to me about his "beautiful" son who was only twelve days old. Although most fathers live with the mother of at least one of their children, some describe their experiences as nonresident or single fathers. Some fathers are homeless. Others are stay-at-home dads. I spoke with eighty-seven men who collectively were raised in at least twenty-one different states or countries and who currently live in one of sixteen states, representing every major region of the United States, with the majority residing in Florida.[10] Including biological, step, and adopted children, these fathers talked about 134 sons and 93 daughters.

I lean heavily on fathers to help me construct an image of how they personally navigate the health matrix as men, coparents, and fathers. In doing so, I can only speculate about how their children or partners actually feel about their experiences independent of what the fathers share with me. However, "children's voices" enter my book when I have the fathers reflect on their childhood experiences in the health matrix. They describe their perceptions as children and their early as well as more recent interactions with their parents, extended kin, and others in the community.

I also share stories from an assortment of fifteen health care professionals who work with kids in home-based programs, private practices, clinics, and in various hospital units. Their candid talk tempers what fathers say they do with and for their children in health care settings and at home. The professionals sometimes comment on fathers' lack of involvement and offer ideas on what might be done to get men more productively involved in their children's health care. Few, however, have channeled their energies to advocate for more active father involvement in their health care practices. In fact, it was striking to me that so many had given so little thought to how dads fit into their children's health care matrix.[11] I hope to inspire more pediatric health care professionals to reach out to fathers and find ways to help them become stronger advocates for their children's well-being.

My approach to interviewing fathers and health care professionals is informed by both my professional training as a social scientist and my experiences as a man who has fathered two sons during decidedly different historical eras, life stages, household contexts, and financial circumstances.[12]

No doubt my experiential wisdom about the health matrix would have been even richer had I also fathered a daughter. Even though I can't manufacture the experience of fathering a daughter, I can and do explore other fathers' stories about how they perceive and interact with their daughters along a full range of health, fitness, and well-being issues.

PERSONAL REFLECTIONS

I distinctly recall how my fitness mentality colored my style of fathering not long after Phoenix's birth. Phoenix had a basketball in his crib before he could pronounce "ball," and he was shooting hoops and dunking routinely on a plastic goal before he could string words together intelligibly. Not surprisingly, once he became a toddler I made a point of buying him the typical sporting gear for the major sports. I also registered him for his first official soccer team, the Lightning Bolts, when he was barely three. I even said yes to a new house purchase partly because it had two and a half acres of land for a child to roam and run. I altered part of the land so that it now supports a fifty-yard field with soccer goals that also serves us well for football, baseball, kickball, dodgeball, and chase games.

Throughout my second stint at fathering, my greater maturity and a flexible work schedule have afforded me plenty of opportunities to promote Phoenix's health and to care for him. Now I have a chance to be the attentive dad who is available and willing to make and attend health appointments, deal with medical emergencies, devote time to investigating car-seat purchases, create food shopping rituals with an educational tone, coach my son's athletic teams, and train him for his triathlons.

Not all fathers (or mothers) have similar "free" time or the financial means to invest in their children. My earlier experience of being a resident working-class teenage father and then, beginning at age twenty-two, a nonresident out-of-state dad opened my eyes to how life conditions can hinder a father's involvement. Back then, my circumstances restricted my options for imparting my values on health and fitness to Scott, my elder son, who turned thirty-nine in 2015. Once I became a nonresident dad, I saw Scott in the summer for three or four weeks and occasionally for a few days at other times during the year. I was largely out of touch with his day-to-day health needs for most of the year, and I never met any of the health care professionals who saw him after he turned four. I've vowed not to miss out on the key opportunities to interact with pediatric professionals and advocate for Phoenix.

The circumstances with Scott were less than ideal for me to introduce him consistently and slowly to my views of healthy eating. Indeed, a major source of tension pitted my health-conscious demands with his more carefree desires for junk food—especially sugary cereals. Ironically, despite our limited and somewhat contentious exchanges during his youth, Scott is now quick to scrutinize food labels and is particular about what he gives his children to eat and drink. He keeps current on the latest nutritional trends and controversies and is better versed than I in the debates about gluten-free diets, food additives, supplements, herbs, and more. Perhaps he was paying attention as a kid after all.

Scott shared some of his adult insights with me one summer when Phoenix and I visited him as part of an 810-mile road trip to a national triathlon competition in Ohio. Beyond getting long overdue face time with Scott, I was able to execute my plan to have my two sons do their first joint running session. An unexpected twist to our family health matrix occurred in Scott's kitchen after the run when he confronted me about the low-fat peanut butter I had packed to make sandwiches for Phoenix and me on our trip. I had been health conscious in my selection, but Scott gave me a quick lecture on the negatives of rapeseed oil, encouraging me to use his organic peanut butter instead, which I did. When I returned home, I jumped on the Internet to learn more about my son's admonition.[13] While reading the mixed assessments of rapeseed oil, I smiled, thinking about how my older son had stepped in to help me and his little brother. In the meantime, I've started to purchase a different kind of peanut butter. My exchange with Scott also reminded me that parent-child relationships are often reciprocal in their effects. Children of varying ages can directly and indirectly influence how their dads and moms approach health and fitness.

A number of the stories dads shared with me about their early upbringing and their own fathering echo my own experiences. But recollections of poverty, addiction, child abuse, neglect, prison time, chronically poor health, and more are foreign to anything I have confronted as a man or father. For many readers, the tragic stories chronicled in this book will put into perspective the nature of the "not-so-bad" circumstances faced by many resident middle-class fathers of "typical" children.

THE MEN'S HEALTH MOVEMENT

When it comes to health and fitness, we live in a uniquely polarized era of good and bad. Today, millions of young and not so young men are every bit as conscientious about their physical and mental well-being as I am. A small subset of men are likely to see me as a slacker when it comes to my fitness regimen and personal health care.

Whether it is highly competitive white-collar professionals who train extensively for triathlons, or blue-collar guys who religiously commit to working out and playing city league or pickup basketball and soccer games at local gyms and parks, or men from different walks of life who exercise on a regular but more modest scale, plenty of adult men are committed to recreational forms of exercise. According to the 2014 National Health Interview Survey of the noninstitutionalized civilian population of the United States, 67 percent of 18- to 24-year-old men and almost 53 percent of 25- to 64-year-old men met the 2008 federal physical activity guidelines for aerobic activity through leisure-time aerobic activity.[14] Another national survey covering the period from 2001 to 2009 reveals a slight increase in the percentage (49.7 to 53.3) of adult men who did five or more days of thirty or more minutes of moderate physical activity, or vigorous physical activity for twenty or more minutes three or more days per week. Complementary trends can be seen in the increasing percentage of men, including many fathers, who are pursuing endurance events such as triathlons.[15]

Other good news is that, as fathers and coaches, men are quicker now to acknowledge the dangers related to concussions that stem from athletic events and recreational play. To their credit, men have slowly become more attentive to their own and young people's brain health. These patterns reflect the larger trend for professional sports organizations and players to take head injuries more seriously.[16] The trend's most symbolic event occurred in 2013, when the National Football League reached a $765 million settlement with the more than 4,500 former football players who had sued the league for being negligent in how it managed their risks of head trauma.[17] The lasting significance of this event was reinforced by the 2015 movie *Concussion* starring Will Smith, who plays Dr. Bennet Omalu, the forensic pathologist who first identified chronic traumatic encephalopathy (CTE) in former professional football players and fought the NFL when it tried to suppress his research.

In an age of greater public awareness about posttraumatic stress disorder (PTSD) and depression, one national study shows that in 1998 about 1.47 of every 100 men sought outpatient help for depression in the United States, a figure that had increased slightly, to 2.12, by 2007.[18] Although it appears that men today are a bit more likely than their counterparts from earlier generations to seek counseling to deal with substance addictions as well as relationship and family issues, they still are not nearly as likely as women to visit a physician. According to surveys sponsored by the Agency for Healthcare Research and Quality (AHRQ), about 57 percent of men visited a doctor within the past year, whereas 74 percent of women did.[19] Trend data indicate that despite the promising upward trend in the proportion of men reporting a physician's office visit between 1995 and 2009, the pattern was reversed in 2010.[20]

In recent years, the AHRQ has partnered with different stakeholders to launch ad campaigns designed to encourage men to be more attentive to their health and to seek preventive screenings. In 2008, the sports network ESPN enlisted the services of prominent sports broadcasters, including Jim Rome, Mike Golic, Mike Greenberg, the late Scott Stuart, and others to reach out to viewers in creative ways.[21] Other provocative public service announcements for TV, radio, and print were created in 2010 to entice or guilt men into getting more preventive checkups.[22] One such ad tried to get men's attention with the message, "This year thousands of men will die from stubbornness." Another notable education campaign, "Drive for Five," was introduced in September of 2012 as part of a partnership between Abbott (now AbbVie), a pharmaceutical company focused on educating men about health, and the Men's Health Network (MHN).[23] This education and health awareness project encourages men to pay attention to high cholesterol, high blood pressure, high blood sugar, high PSA (prostate-specific antigen), and low testosterone.

The success of popular magazines like *Men's Health* and *Men's Fitness* attests to the increasingly pervasive public discourse that encourages men to be more responsible in taking care of their bodies and minds. Boasting circulations of 1.9 million and more than 585,000 respectively, the magazines clearly reach a substantial number of men.[24] However, do these magazines simply reflect a shift in some men's consciousness, or have they actually altered men's orientation toward healthy living? Perhaps it's a bit of both. At the very least, the magazines seem to mark a new, more progressive era in how men relate to their bodies and construct their identities.

Men receive varying levels of emotional support from their network of close friends and family, but fathers of young children today are, generally speaking, in a better position than their fathers were at a comparable stage in their lives to attend to their own physical and emotional well-being. As a result, men are gradually becoming less dependent on a mother, grandmother, wife, or romantic partner to monitor their health care, even though many still do.[25] Armed with this newfound confidence, the most recent generation of fathers is likely to see that having an active and open mind about their children's health needs is the new normal.

INSTITUTIONAL HEALTH INITIATIVES

Organized efforts to promote men's and fathers' health are taking place globally.[26] Government initiatives in the United States, Australia, Europe, and elsewhere have sought to transform men's orientation to their own health.[27] In some instances these health-based initiatives are loosely tied to broader social policies designed to recognize, understand, and promote fathers' contributions to their families. As recently as 2011, the United Nations took stock of the policy options available to governments that could alter fathers' involvement in, and contributions to, family life.[28] In *Men in Families and Family Policy in a Changing World,* the UN focused both on how fathering influences men's health and on how fathers can influence their children's well-being, especially in the context of disabilities. The UN recommended strategies to promote men's caregiving by expanding paternity leave, offering more flexible work options, altering family laws to promote joint custody, developing public school initiatives to offer more life skills courses for boys, and training public health personnel to encourage men's involvement in care work. In addition, a call was made to "encourage men to participate in maternal and child care, including during childbirth and in all matters involving reproductive and sexual health."[29] These recommendations speak to the stark reality: the changing demography of fatherhood and women's labor market activity have transformed the larger context in which men make choices and are involved in families.

MenCare is a global multimedia campaign that promotes fatherhood and men's caregiving. This initiative sponsors a wide range of programs designed to help fathers, mothers, and children. Its mission is to "promote men's involvement as equitable, non-violent fathers and caregivers in order to achieve family well-being and gender equality."[30] As of July 2015 it was active in Africa, Asia Pacific, Europe and Central Asia, and Latin America.

In the United States, nonprofit organizations like the Men's Health Network, founded in 1993, have moved men's health issues into the national spotlight. MHN's mission is to "reach men and their families where they live, work, play, and pray with health prevention messages and tools, screening programs, educational materials, advocacy opportunities, and patient navigation." This organization includes physicians, researchers, public health workers, and other health professionals. With publications like the *Blueprint for Men's Health: A Guide to a Healthy Lifestyle*, MHN offers men practical knowledge and resources to become more conscientious about their health. It provides advocates with an effective platform to encourage men's and boys' health. More recently, MHN was one of nine cosponsoring organizations that spearheaded the 2012 Dialogue on Men's Health Conference. This conference generated a report on the health and wellness of American boys and men issued by the Men's Health Braintrust.[31] As the pro-health message finds its way into traditionally masculine settings such as work and sports, men are likely to grow more comfortable assessing their own health needs and taking care of them.

Unfortunately, despite some modest overtures in the United States and elsewhere, relatively little is being done to connect issues concerning fathers' and children's health.[32] A critical next step for government and nonprofit organizations is to promote more clearly how the health of men, as fathers, is related to their children's health. As I mention in the preface, in the fall of 2014 I went public with a website, *Dads & Kids: Health & Fitness Talk*, and a companion Facebook page to accentuate the ties between fathers' and children's health. These outlets underscore the value of designing resources to help dads contribute positively to their children's well-being. While emphasizing the everyday realties facing fathers who come from diverse backgrounds and a range of family-health circumstances, my Internet-based projects spotlight the four partnerships outlined earlier (father-child, father-coparent, father–non-family members, and community organizations' interactions). I show how these partnerships affect fathers' and children's options to leave a healthy imprint on each other's lives.

The positive patterns that document men's improving health profile are offset by several undesirable trends in men's self-reports spanning the period from 1999 to 2012 that may negatively influence child outcomes.[33] Information collected from the National Health and Nutritional Examination Surveys and the National State of Obesity report show that whereas 27.5 percent of men were obese (body mass index [BMI] of 30 to 99.8) in 1999–2000, that figure jumped to 36.5 percent in 2011–2012. BMI scores in the 20–25 range are considered healthy; those below 20 indicate a person may be underweight and scores above 25 indicate a person may be overweight. That almost 17 percent of male children age two to nineteen are obese compared to 14 percent a decade earlier suggests that high obesity rates for adult men are likely to continue unless a drastic change occurs. For years we have known that kids who are obese have a very high probability of being overweight as adults.[34] In recent years, researchers in the UK and Australia have shown that the BMI for fathers is an important predictor of high BMI values for children and children's greater likelihood of being obese.[35]

One of the main concerns about childhood obesity is that it often leads to serious health consequences such as diabetes and cardiovascular disease in adulthood. The data reveal more bad news: as of 1999, 5.9 percent of men said that they, at some point in their lives, had been told that they had diabetes, whereas 8.8 percent made the same claim in 2009. In 1999, 23 percent said they had been told by a health professional sometime in their lives that they had high blood pressure. Almost 30 percent of men gave the same response when interviewed a decade later. The percentage of men reporting that they had been told that their blood cholesterol was high jumped from 29.6 percent in 1999 to nearly 40 percent in 2009.

Despite these undesirable patterns, trend data offer one piece of good news: the percentage of adult men eighteen years of age and older currently smoking declined from 23.9 in 2005 to 20.5 in 2013.[36] This trend portends a possible reduction in the proportion of children who experiment with smoking and develop an addiction to it.[37]

Young and not so young men still disproportionately engage in all sorts of risk-taking behaviors at high rates. Compared to women, men are more likely to smoke, eat fatty foods, drink and drive, use guns, play violent sports, and not get enough sleep. Men are also less likely to get routine physicals or seek professional attention for more serious matters. These trends remind me of a story a former student shared about her grandfather: while working at home with a nail gun, he accidentally shot a nail through his hand, yanked the nail out, wrapped his hand in a cloth, and continued to work for the rest of the day before seeking medical treatment later that night. This grandfather is not alone. Numerous hard-core "manly men" are still out there; they must either see blood gushing from their body in order to consider receiving medical treatment, or have persistent suicidal thoughts in order to consider seeking counseling advice.

All of these health and fitness patterns—the good and the bad—are closely tied to financial resources. Exercising regularly, eating well, having access to adequate health care, being physically safe, and avoiding environmental health risks are bigger challenges for people living in urban slums or public housing. Life is also rough for those grappling with extreme rural poverty. The health matrix for fathers and their kids is deeply rooted in systems of poverty and privilege, as well as institutionalized racism. Clearly, far more than DNA, personality, and motivation shape people's relative health risks and practical access to health care.

For decades, numerous writers affiliated with the field of men's studies have critically evaluated the gender gap in health outcomes by exploring how conventional expressions of a masculine identity affect men's health- and fitness-related decisions and experiences.[38] These commentators highlight the negative consequences boys and men often encounter when they try to honor a code of manly conduct that curbs their health consciousness and self-care. Many point to how men's lower life expectancy is not simply a matter of physiological differences between males and females; rather, they suggest that a web of social forces accounts for men's shorter life span. These conditions affect how men experience and respond to the challenges associated with depression, prostate cancer, binge drinking, violence, heart disease, and more.

The crux of this line of thinking says that boys, unfortunately, are taught from a very early age to be tough, stoic risk takers who should endure lots of discomfort and pain without complaint. Boys are also told to keep their vulnerabilities and emotional troubles under wraps. As boys grow into men cultural expectations remain much the same, leaving too many men with the impression that seeking medical attention is a sign of weakness. In addition, many men are encouraged to believe that their mission in life is to become an economic provider for their family, even if this means working at jobs that jeopardize their health.

In recent years, gender scholars, including health social scientists, recognize that masculine identity can be produced in diverse ways and is shaped by men's circumstances related to age, social class, sexual orientation, race and ethnicity, and cultural background. A common theme woven throughout the literature connecting masculinity and health is that the things that negatively affect some men's health are intertwined with social realities that tend to favor men in general. For example, the economic world has historically provided men with more, and higher-paying, work opportunities, but these positions often lead to physical and mental health problems.

Those alarmed by how a patriarchal society and gender norms affect men's health typically support a profeminist stance on men's relations with women and other men. This progressive agenda, with its emphasis on gender equity, encourages men to take a more active role in domestic affairs, including child care. It also challenges men to develop supportive, emotionally authentic relationships with other men.

THE CHANGING LANDSCAPE OF MASCULINITY AND FATHERING

Public perceptions of good fathering have evolved in recent decades thanks to expanding views about what constitutes acceptable displays of manhood and masculinity, the changing demographic profile of families, media portrayals, grassroots activities, academic and popular press publications, and social policies.

The dramatic shift in gender relations in the United States over the last fifty years has created new opportunities and expectations for boys, men, and fathers alike. As women's options for tailoring their work and family life have grown, men's perceptions of and experiences in these areas has changed as well. More men now align themselves with ideals consistent with a profeminist approach, but aside from social activists or those like myself who work in the gender studies field, most don't adopt the feminist label. Yet, in practical terms, these men are profeminist partly because they see their masculine identities in a new light, are willing to speak out against domestic violence, and believe it's their responsibility, perhaps privilege, to pursue gender equity in its many forms, including caring directly for their children's daily needs.[39] Compared to earlier generations of dads, who spent less time with their kids, they also voice greater frustration about work-family conflicts.[40] Those who are straight tend to maintain a style of partnership with their romantic partners that differs considerably from the model used by their grandparents and parents. As these "modern men" redefine how they see and relate to their partners—and women more generally—they are transforming their approach to fathering. Moreover, what some have termed the "new fatherhood" is a product of the larger shift in gender relations that the women's movement inspired and that the men's movement activities, which followed, made more salient to men.

Today, being a good financial provider, but little else, is no longer enough to be a good father. Fathers are expected to be there both physically and emotionally for their kids. But it's not just the "father-as-wallet" mentality that is being questioned. Compared to their own fathers and grandfathers, contemporary fathers are actually doing more hands-on caregiving with their children, especially if they live together.[41]

Dads' increasing hands-on care arises partly out of necessity as more families navigate time management issues in dual-earner households. However, this trend also mirrors the changing cultural messages that give dads more latitude to express themselves as manly men beyond the scope of exclusively being their children's provider and protector. Granted, many men still see much of domestic labor and child care as mainly women's work. However, the images of what "real men" are able to do with and for their kids have evolved to include more nurturing, health-based care.

The shift in how fathers should relate to their kids is also connected to how men in recent years have been given more leeway to adopt what has been traditionally perceived to be a more feminine style of self-care. Recall that a key objective of the men's health movement is to transform the way boys and men think about and care for their own health needs. As rigid expectations about manly stoicism and indifference to health needs give way to healthier norms about men's physical and emotional self-care, contemporary dads have a unique opportunity to become healthier role models and advisors for their kids. In the abstract, this seems ideal. In reality, men's actual experiences may lag behind the cultural prescriptions that encourage men to embrace a healthier lifestyle. This disconnect is most obvious for low-income men, whose ability to adopt a healthier lifestyle is more likely to be hampered by financial constraints as well as by cultural pressures of a traditional brand of masculinity that dismiss self-care as feminine.

In *Nurturing Dads: Social Initiatives for Contemporary Fatherhood*, I describe with my coauthor Kevin Roy how progressive initiatives on various fronts can help transform the model of the exclusive breadwinner dad to one that champions the ideal dad as engaged and nurturing. Drawing on interviews with several hundred men, mostly fathers, we argue that a wide range of public and private initiatives should take into account the complex, everyday realities that define contemporary fathers' lives.

The demographic landscape of fathering has shifted; it now features relatively large numbers of single dads, stay-at-home dads, nonresident dads, gay dads, dads with children from different mothers, stepdads, immigrant dads, dads of internationally adopted children, and more. Despite its less than modern depiction of women's professional aptitudes, the Emmy-award-winning TV sitcom *Modern Family*, which premiered in 2009, does an excellent job of depicting the increasing diversity of American families. For instance, actors Eric Stonestreet and Jesse Tyler Ferguson play a gay couple who adopt a baby girl from Vietnam. Apart from such media influences, statistics also help frame the story of family change. From 1960 to 2011 the number of single fathers increased from 297,000 to almost 2.7 million; between 1989 and 2010 the number of fathers who were at home with their children for any reason doubled from 1.1 to 2.2 million, with the number declining slightly since the official end of the recession. Whereas only 5 percent of stay-at-home dads in 1989 reported that they were not working primarily because they were caring for their home or family, 21 percent gave this reason in 2012.[42]

Many fathers face new and challenging life circumstances. This stems partly from the changing landscape in which more mothers are working— and in working more have less time to devote to domestic life. Such a kaleidoscope of conditions breeds diverse family networks and a maze of interpersonal relations. Additionally, many more fathers are experiencing personal conflict between work and family obligations, casting this tension in a new, more critical light.[43]

Some highly engaged dads are actually experiencing less stress, however. These men, referred to as "superdads" by sociologist Gayle Kaufman, see their caregiver role as more important than being a breadwinner.[44] They want to maximize their time with their kids and they "*deliberately adjust their work lives to fit their family lives,* rather than vice versa."[45] This pattern reflects what most women in the labor force have been obligated to do for years.

Overall, the changing landscape of fathering has produced mixed results for fathers and their families. Some cultural and social developments enhance fathers' ability to shape their children's orientation toward health and fitness, whereas others constrain that ability. As families and households become increasingly diverse and fluid, the family bargains men strike in the name of coparenting look different as well. For example, compared to a resident biological father, a nonresident or stepdad who happens to be a vegan or vegetarian may have little sway in how his children manage their eating habits when the children live with and take their dietary cues from the meat-eating mom.

Some family arrangements clearly affect the extent to which—or even whether—fathers are involved in their children's health- and fitness-related matters. For example, if a father only sees his middle-school child one weekend a month, he may struggle to establish a clear set of nutritional and mealtime routines. A limited child visitation schedule too often fosters a "Disney Dad" style of fathering in which fathers take their kids to fun places and eat out.[46] Whether it is actually a Disney theme park, or a baseball game, a movie, McDonald's, or Chuck E. Cheese, these sites typically produce unhealthy eating excursions. So too, fathers who seldom see their children may look to avoid conflict and cave in to requests for unhealthy snacks, sodas, and meals high in fat content and loaded with calories. In contrast, if the father secures full-time residential custody of the child he will be better positioned to persuade his child to be a vegetarian or carnivore; push his philosophy on sickness, vitamins, herbs, medicine, and fitness; and enforce or discourage health and safety practices based on his policies for the use of sunscreen, helmets, seatbelts, hand sanitizer, and curfews. And for better or worse, the resident father is also better positioned to become the attentive parent who coaches his kids in their youth sports.[47]

Whether fathers share a home with their children all, some, or none of the time, a father-child bond is commonly expressed in one of four basic forms: behavioral, cognitive, emotional, and spiritual or ethical. Bonds are "enduring sentiments that motivate a father to want to be involved with his child and to embrace certain parental obligations while committing his time, energy, and resources to enhance his child's well-being."[48] For both fathers and children alike, strong bonds foster a sense of being part of an "us" or sharing a "we" feeling. The affinity symbolizes a degree of reciprocal trust. Children who experience this we-ness may better understand motives, their own as well as those of others. They may be more willing to see their fathers as making good-faith efforts to respond to their developmentally appropriate needs. In other words, when children respect and trust their fathers they are more likely to embrace their fathers' healthy messages: to exercise, eat vegetables, avoid drugs, get proper sleep, wear a bike helmet, and so forth. If children are receptive, dads may be more comfortable staying on message or occasionally reinforcing it. Dads will certainly feel less stress in doing so if their children appear to entertain their fathers' comments open-mindedly and sometimes alter their behavior accordingly. If children feel included in the process of carving out a healthy lifestyle with their fathers' guidance, they may develop a sense of ownership and control when they make healthy choices. On the flip side, reciprocal trust can lead children to mirror their fathers' unhealthy habits of eating poorly, drinking alcohol, smoking cigarettes, driving fast, and playing with guns.

Fathers' family circumstances can also affect how people process images of the "good father." These images reflect how fathers bond with their children and what each prioritizes. Because "unconventional" families are quite common, large numbers of fathers and children must navigate poorly defined family terrain to achieve affinity. Single dads, nonresident fathers, stepdads, and gay fathers grapple with family circumstances that are more fluid and subject to negotiation than those typically found in two-parent, resident heterosexual families. Fathers living in unconventional arrangements can be effective messengers for healthy living, but their road to success tends to be less clearly mapped and direct.

The shifting landscape of fathering also means that, compared to earlier cohorts, more kids today use a different lens to view and judge their family experiences. With greater access to modern media, kids are less sheltered and more street smart. As a result, they are better positioned to understand, shape, and confront their fathers. Today more than ever, children are not simply vessels that parents fill with life lessons. In the Internet age, several key strokes can provide computer-literate kids "evidence" to either refute or confirm adult claims. Kids, directly and indirectly, can challenge their fathers' unhealthy ways or support their healthy choices.

FATHERING IN AN AGE OF SPECIAL NEEDS

Public sentiment that nurturance should be a more central piece of "good fathering" complements the growing awareness that more and more fathers have children with special needs. The "special needs" label refers to a wide range of diagnoses that hinder a child's ability to perform certain tasks. Generally speaking, special needs are grouped into behavioral, developmental, learning, medical, and mental health categories. As specific conditions such as ADHD, autism, asthma, learning disabilities, and obesity have become more prevalent in recent years, fathers increasingly find themselves in a position to address their children's real and perceived limitations.

Unfortunately, medical and social service professionals have focused less attention on fathers than on mothers in families with special needs. The general public and medical community have, however, slowly acknowledged that fathers can and sometimes do help their kids manage their poor health. To their credit, researchers have recently started to look into how fathers perceive and care for their chronically ill children.[49] Still, a number of studies show that in the case of families with chronically ill children, fathers often see themselves as the "forgotten" parent and may not receive adequate social and emotional support.[50]

Just as the diversity in family structure affects fathers' opportunities to interact with their "typical" children, being part of an unconventional family form can alter the fathering landscape for those raising children with special needs. For various reasons—including fathers' work schedules and lax caregiving motivation—health care professionals and related staff are challenged to incorporate fathers into the familial support and treatment team. Although difficulties can arise irrespective of the family arrangement, split households often create the worst friction and most notable logistical problems.

On the whole, when I interview men with children who have special needs I sense that most are intimately involved in caring for their children. My admiration for the dads is tempered, though, when I listen to various pediatric health care providers describe their encounters with families. Reports depict many fathers as being less informed and less involved than mothers. One pediatric nurse practitioner, Yvonne, who had two years of experience overseeing a nursing home-care program for families with chronically ill children in an urban setting, paints a very bleak picture. "In the home care field, I honestly can't recall ever seeing a dad on a regular basis. It was *always* the mothers." She couldn't recall having any significant contact with the children's fathers. Even though fathers lived in many of the households, they were not as emotionally or practically invested in their children's care.

Given children's vulnerability, the public and the medical community typically frame the special needs world by targeting children's limitations and needs. Of course kids are not the only family members who struggle with health-related problems. But far less attention has been given to the trials and tribulations of fathers (and mothers) who are trying to raise children despite their own chronic illnesses and debilitating conditions.[51]

I spoke with a number of fathers who fit this description—men hampered by post-traumatic stress disorder (PTSD) and post-concussion syndrome (PCS) caused by deployments to Iraq and Afghanistan, MS, blindness, Crohn's disease, diabetes, ADHD, autism, limb amputation, heart disease, mental illnesses like schizophrenia and bipolar disorder, as well as by conditions more likely to be viewed as self-inflicted, such as drug and alcohol addictions. Fathers' health issues owing to bad luck, bad DNA, or bad personal choices can compromise the level and quality of their interactions with their children. Unfortunately, few initiatives have been designed specifically to help fathers or mothers deal with chronic health problems so they can be more productive parents and become better advocates for their children's health. I trust the perspective I offer here will nudge critical stakeholders to pay more attention in their programming to get fathers more involved.

GAINING PERSPECTIVE

Fathers deal not only with chronic conditions but also with intermittent or isolated events that adversely affect both their quality of health and their ability to interact as they would like to with their children. I gained insights firsthand about this after having surgeries a year apart for a torn medial meniscus in my right knee and a herniated disc in my lower back when Phoenix was four and five years old, respectively. My recoveries from these surgeries, and the debilitating troubles I experienced prior to them, significantly reduced my mobility for months. Much to my dismay, I had to modify my hands-on, athletic style of fathering for each surgery. No longer could I coach my son's soccer team. I postponed our bike rides and my quest to set him free from training wheels. Our one-on-one kickball and football competitions turned into walking, stand-up affairs, at least for me. I watched him stretch singles into home runs as I labored in the field. I experimented with altering the distance between the bases to level the "playing field," but my tinkering produced a poetic injustice. While greater spacing limited his home runs, I was less likely to reach first base safely when I kicked. In our football sessions, Phoenix was forced into full-time receiver duty. Whatever throwing he did was to a stationary target—me. Pool time was skipped entirely. And on doctor's orders, especially those that came from my back surgeon, I was not permitted to lift Phoenix or throw him in the air. We put on hold special tossing gestures that have for years spiced up our celebratory, hello, and bonding rituals.

Although I tried to reconfigure our play time as best I could, my physical setbacks disrupted my style of fathering. Phoenix, like most young five-year-olds, occasionally morphed into a bratty combatant when my limitations got the better of him. He was frustrated that we had to abandon our typically intense and running style of sports play. His disappointment, in turn, rattled me—I felt old, irrelevant, washed up. In years past, I had coped reasonably well when I was forced to give up competitive sports with my peers, but now I was unable even to hold my own with a five-year-old.

When I redirected my self-pity, I realized my life circumstances paled in comparison to the daily struggles many fathers face. Fortunately, I gained perspective by mulling over stories like Edward's, who described his lifestyle transition, which he traced back to his mid-thirties when he was diagnosed with MS. He gradually went from being a physically fit father of two young boys and a successful, hardworking physician to a disabled father of young men and a prematurely retired doctor in his mid-fifties living with the reality that his life would forever be affected by the disease. Confined to a scooter for the past several years, Edward was the first dad I personally interviewed for this book. At one point, sitting poolside on his back porch one morning, I listened intently to Edward share what life was like when he was forty-one and coaching his youngest son's recreational basketball team.

> I remember I had a noticeable limp when I was coaching . . . and I'm thinking, "I'm glad I'm doing this now because I won't be able to do this soon." I knew what was coming, but you'd have to go from defense to offense and I would limp and throw the ball in and you know when [older son] was the same age I could dunk a basketball and I could play full-court games, so, my health slowly deteriorated as my kids grew up, but we [wife and Edward] did not want them to think that Dad was any different, and that we had a sad, sick household, so, you know, I try, to this day, not to dwell. You know, we're all going to live and we're all going to die, the body gets old and you know I had a fairly good run as being an active, biking, basketball playing, you know, softball league, type guy.

His story resonated with me because Edward and I shared much in common as former competitive basketball players and I had just started my own journey of coaching Phoenix's soccer and basketball teams. Despite his current circumstances, or perhaps because of them, Edward anchors his story to what he perceives to be the good news. Edward is thankful that the full, debilitating effects of MS had progressed slowly enough so as not to eliminate completely his ability to create some action-oriented memories with both of his sons. I sensed that Edward takes special delight in once having had the ability to run, jump, and dunk. He passed on his love for basketball to his sons.

For now, having learned how to adjust to being an engaged father who just happens to have MS, he is most shaken by his inability to be the kind of son he would like to be to his elderly father who lives out of state. "One of my biggest sorrows is that I can't see my dad . . . he can't fly and I can't fly anymore because it's such a nightmare. If the plane is delayed and I can't get to the bathroom and it's so anxiety-provoking that I just can't do it."

We didn't talk about it, but I fear Edward is destined to feel the emotional anguish of not being able to visit loved ones who live far away for the rest of his life. In the years ahead, how will Edward's travel restrictions affect the way he experiences being a family man to his twenty-six- and twenty-year-old sons, who will likely start their own families? Surely his experiences with any grandchildren who may someday come into his life will be restricted in ways he had not imagined prior to his diagnosis. Although his able-bodied wife has been quite supportive throughout his illness, Edward is likely to experience some envy when he sees his wife interacting physically with their children and potential grandchildren in ways that he can't.

Edward's story is a good reminder that the journey to becoming and being a father is shaped by all sorts of cultural forces, family dynamics, and personal circumstances. Throughout our lives, we are exposed as fathers to diverse messages from diverse sources. Some directly, others indirectly, influence our approach to health, fitness, and well-being for ourselves and our children. My own life-long affinity for sports, nurtured years ago by the collective mind of a small working-class town where a boy's athletic prowess profoundly affected his social status, remains etched in my psyche as a man and as a father. It continues to shape my understanding of how the health matrix frames my experiences and those of others.

My exchanges with fathers and pediatric health care professionals afford me unique opportunities to compare and assess how my life as a man and father fits into the health matrix. With each conversation I sharpen my perspective as to what kind of man I've been, what kind of man I am, and what kind of man I hope to be. Similarly, and perhaps more importantly, these talks force me to reflect on what kind of father I've been, what kind of father I am, and what kind of father I want to be. Others, I hope, will experience a similar type of personal growth when they reflect on the stories I share in this book. The stories, when studied collectively, reveal how social forces frame the health matrix for all sorts of fathers and children.

At times, challenging circumstances in the form of limited finances, health problems, or coparental discord restrict fathers' ability to be as health conscious as they might otherwise be for themselves or their children. Yet some fathers find creative and inspiring ways to overcome their life obstacles and take an active role in promoting their kids' health and fitness while modeling a healthy lifestyle for them. And although the stories in this book focus on men's and fathers' lives, girls and women—most notably the daughters and coparenting mothers—play a prominent role in how the fathers experience the health matrix.

2 ❧ FROM BEING A BOY TO BECOMING A DADDY

SOME OF MY FONDEST childhood memories include exploring the dense woods around my house in western Pennsylvania. Unfortunately, my discovery time was limited, especially in the summer, because I honored Mom's warnings to avoid the poison ivy that gave me itchy misery. I still did my fair share of navigating creek rocks, climbing trees, digging trenches, scaling imposing hillsides, running the paths, and penetrating a little deeper into the uncharted land from time to time. Much of my preteen and early teen free time was spent outside playing ball in the neighborhood yards, driveways, and streets, sometimes with Dad, but mostly with three older boys, Keith, Robin, and Wendy. Time passed effortlessly. Play was never stopped because I was tired or bored—rather the dinner bell rang or darkness fell.

Those vivid images of nature and my love for sports raced through my mind as I sat in my office listening to Mark, now forty-five, reminisce about his magnificent childhood adventure in the rural Northwest. Mark's face took on a boyish look as he reflected back to his preteen years, when he spent most of his free time with his younger brother outdoors in the "open pasture land and national forest across the river." He says, "There was a river out back, we swam, we were playing some sport, football, basketball, baseball principally. . . . we had friends that lived a couple miles away and [when] we wanted to go see them we just walked, so it was a life of sort of constant athletic engagement and constant outdoor physical activity." Mark recalls having a "ton" of outside "imaginative free play."

When Mark took me deeper into his childhood memories, I thought of one of my favorite books, *The Last Child in the Woods*, by Richard Louv. As a child advocate, Louv's mission for nearly a decade has been to challenge parents and mentors of children to confront how our fascination with technology and our children's penchant for being "plugged in" has resulted in what he unofficially calls "nature-deficit disorder."[1] Louv believes that the declining mental and physical health of children, along with their behavioral problems, stems in no small measure from children's growing disconnect from nature.

For Mark, and a number of the other fathers who shared their stories with me, being the type of father who encourages his child to connect with nature is often rooted in fond childhood memories of time spent playing and working in the outdoors. The outdoor time together is also seen as valuable because it creates bonding opportunities for fathers and children. Brent talks about how being outdoors together helped him develop stronger relationships with his daughter and son.

> I think being outside and in the outdoors, created much more of a bond because when you're indoors, you're watching TV or playing a video game, or doing something like that, you're not really communicating. When you're outside and you're looking at stuff, "Hey, wow did you see that little frog, did you see that ant, what is this, you know, let's go climb this tree," you're, helpin' each other, you're doin' things together, you're talking more, so I think it absolutely made our relationship much stronger, much deeper, I think it made the bond, I don't think it would be as tight as it would be now, if it wasn't for the fact that we spent a lot of time outside.

Beyond his imaginary outdoors play, Mark also participated in lots of organized sports in his childhood and teen years. He recognizes that his dad, despite his busy schedule, made a point of introducing him and his little brother to various sports, devoting many hours to playing with them out-side. During those early years there was a natural, unspoken rhythm to his life and being healthy. "I go to the gym now, but I was fit then because that was my life, it was just what we did, we thought of it as play, even when it was organized, it was part of our identity in a certain sense and not some-thing that we thought of as part [of a workout regimen]."

Having plenty of time and opportunity to exercise his body as a kid, Mark assumes too that his childhood diet has significantly affected the qual-ity of his life throughout the years:

> I attribute the fact that I'm not incredibly out of shape because all we did was eat incredibly healthy food. We had an acre-large garden. We had wild black-berry bushes all over; we had three acres; we had a trout stream and salmon stream; in the back we had eighteen apple trees, every kind you could imag-ine, from crab to Granny Smith to you name it. We had plum trees, pear trees, quince trees . . . from that level it was extraordinary, because in the early sev-enties when I was there they talked about the three-acre Eden, they didn't talk about organics, of course it was all organic, my dad shot deer and [so we ate] venison, my mom canned things and we helped her can stuff. There was always the stuff that we grew that we ate fresh. It was just, it was an amazingly healthy lifestyle, basically no soda, little candy.

At eleven, Mark said goodbye to his rural paradise and moved with his family to the urban Northeast. Not only did his family have far less space and money, his parents were not around the house nearly as much. As a result, he and his brother were left to fend for themselves. This often pro-duced poor eating binges. All things considered, though, Mark's quality of life as a child was exceptional, and even his teen years, though relatively less wholesome, were free of any major life or health traumas. Mark's early years gave him solid footing to transition into being a man and a father to his pre-teen daughter, who suffers from Type 1 diabetes, and to his young son.

Tivon, a fifty-five-year-old man who survived a fairly tough and unusual childhood, was not so lucky. He was raised in the public housing projects of New York City during the school year, when he stayed with his father; in the summers he spent time with his grandmother in the rural South. Unfor-tunately, Tivon's father had no interest in nurturing a partnership with him that would enhance his health and fitness. With decades of sadness etched into his eyes, Tivon says, "My father spent more time drinking and partying and my stepmother did not care that much for me. So I was, kind of like, ostracized, you know what I mean. Just pushed aside. Wasn't a lot of time spent as far as trying to teach me how to cope and deal with the streets of New York or how to . . . grow up and deal. So I had to learn on my own and I learned from the streets and came up a very bad kid for a while."

Tivon suffered badly from asthma as a child. He recalls that his aunt's homemade remedy for his breathing problems—his towel-draped head positioned over a heated bowl filled with hot water and a big spoonful of Vick's VapoRub—landed him in the hospital with pneumonia for two months. The adults who watched him restricted his outside play time, regularly forcing him inside when the other kids were engrossed in their games. When he was allowed outside the kids still had him pegged as the sick kid when picking teams: "I don't want you on my team 'cause you can't breathe." He couldn't escape others' judgments, but he persevered and tried to play whenever he could.

At ten he fell off the monkey bars at a playground, cracked his skull badly, was taken to the hospital, and has had frequent headaches for the past forty-five years. Things did not improve with age.

Tivon's teen years were filled with dramatic life challenges, beginning when his father came home one day and discovered that he had messed around with his hair products.

> I remember him telling me to get out of the bed and I remember him grabbing me by the neck. And I was about fourteen, fifteen then, and I got a junior black belt from the state of New York and he slapped me. And I should have known better but I kicked him in the groin and my father picked me up and threw me across the bed into the wall, picked me up again, threw me across the bed, and then he put his knees into my arms and he beat me until I was black and blue in the face, broke my jaw and my nose. My stepmother had to hit him in the head with a hammer to make him stop. That, needless to say—it did traumatize me somewhat.

Not surprisingly, Tivon never returned to his father's house to live. By the following year he was doing cocaine, heroin, and other hard drugs. Tivon's approach to his asthma took a turn for the worse too when he was fifteen, after his cousin of the same age died from an asthma attack.

All my aunts and cousin were saying oh I would be dead and I would be next . . . don't let him go outside, don't let him play. And I'm actually sitting there thinking okay the next asthma attack I have can kill me . . . and three days later after he died . . . at his funeral I was standing there looking at his body, you know viewing his body, I can't breathe, right. And I'm terrified because I'm thinking I'm going to die too . . . I ended up getting swooped up and taken outside and put in the car and whisked away.

During his teen years Tivon ran with a gang until he announced he was leaving. On the spot he had to win his freedom by submitting to a gang beating that left him with bruised ribs, lots of welts and knots, a broken tooth, and split lip. He survived and shortly thereafter enlisted in the service, where he was shot in the knee in a military mission overseas. Troubles with drug and alcohol addiction, violence, prison time, and a range of physical ailments including an ulcer, high blood pressure, diabetes, hepatitis C, bulging disks, and PTSD wrought havoc on his adult life after the service.

The fallout from Tivon's assorted problems extends well beyond his own life. These issues have adversely affected the kind of father he has been to his four children with four different mothers. By all accounts, Tivon has, by choice or circumstance, led an unhealthy life. For much of his life, he has had strained, distant, and ineffective relationships with his children.

GROWING UP

I began my interviews with fathers by asking what their lives were like growing up. I had them focus on their experiences with exercise, sports, diet, illnesses, injuries, as well as their family and social life more generally. How did they spend their time? What did they eat? What did their parents, grandparents, siblings, and other adults do and say that mattered to them? What were their neighborhoods like? How did illnesses, injuries, or physical conditions affect them during their younger years?

Having fathers revisit their youth is important, because long before men become fathers, and often before they even become men, men piece together an outlook on their body, nutrition, interpersonal coping, and fitness, whether they know it or not. Though not destiny, our early views often shape how we live life as men and fathers. The teenage binge drinker too often becomes the adult who continues to abuse alcohol and becomes an alcoholic. The sedentary, obese child too often transitions into an adult who either ignores his obesity or battles weight issues unsuccessfully year after year. The child exposed to domestic violence has a greater chance to experience distress, adjustment problems, depression, and trauma-related symptoms as an adult.[2]

A young boy's orientation toward health and fitness is likely to be rooted in his genetic heritage and physical misfortunes, as well as lessons learned in everyday life. Having a congenital or genetic disorder, or simply a physical predisposition to unhealthy outcomes, can put a boy on course to encounter all sorts of unpleasant and challenging circumstances. The physical realities can also influence how boys eventually, as fathers, see and respond to their own children.

Gerald, a forty-year-old African American single father of a fifteen-year-old boy, had breathing problems in his youth that resulted from a serious case of pneumonia before his second birthday. He struggled to cope with being a small, skinny kid who mistakenly thought he had only one lung—much later he came to realize that only part of his lung had been removed. What he knew for sure as a child was that he tired more quickly than his peers. Gerald assumed his fatigue was caused by his lung condition, but he never told anyone because he feared others would stigmatize him.

In his eyes, whenever his addict father was in the family picture, he was overprotective. He would monitor Gerald's activities and come outside and tell other kids to ease up on him if he felt they were playing too rough with him. These reminders of his frailty may have lowered Gerald's self-esteem. Although protective in this way, the father never talked to Gerald about his family history of high blood pressure and diabetes or discussed his own addiction to drugs.

Gerald has made some modest efforts to be a different kind of father. Despite his own shortcomings—Gerald hasn't been to a physician in close to twenty years and his diet is heavy on fried, fatty foods—he has at least told his son about their family health history and candidly talks to him about the things he did as a kid (being sexually active, drinking) and the problems his father had with drugs. Gerald admits to being quick-tempered and is also mindful of the lingering effects that seeing his father hit his mother have had on him. Last year, Gerald ended his troubled relationship with his long-time cohabiting partner because he did not want to risk having his son witness the same kind of tension that he saw between his own parents when he was younger.

The kind of forward-thinking, protective fathering Gerald describes draws attention to many children's bleak realities. According to a 2008 national survey of 4,549 American children seventeen years of age and younger, 17.9 percent were exposed to intimate partner violence at some point during their lifetime, and 6.6 percent were exposed to that form of violence within the past year.[3] Among the children age 14 to 17, 27.7 reported exposure to intimate partner violence in their lifetime. Studies show that compared to their nonexposed peers, children in violent families tend to exhibit more aggressive and antisocial behavior.[4] Children exposed to domestic violence also experience negative emotional health outcomes similar to those reported by children who are physically abused themselves. Fortunately, Gerald's son may have been saved from the misfortunes that so many children encounter because of the vicious intergenerational cycle of troubled childhoods and violent fathering.

Unlike Gerald, Landen, a twenty-nine-year-old father of two small children, had no issues with domestic violence growing up and no real health worries until he was twelve. Then Landen's knee unexpectedly gave out while he was running wind sprints at a basketball practice. X-rays revealed that he had osteogenic sarcoma—bone cancer that affected his entire patella. In short order, his playful childhood days turned into a sober medical ordeal. He had the lower portion of his leg amputated as part of an unusual, creative surgery. In his words, "They take your knee out and cut about halfway up your femur and of the lower leg, the lower part of the leg, and take all of that out, and then they reconnect your foot 180 degrees backwards, but where your knee would be. So, you use your foot and ankle as a moveable knee joint, but you still have all of the feeling, all of the senses, and movement is all your own."

His divorced parents and entire family rallied around him. According to Landen, although his mother was fond of telling him "mind over matter" as he confronted getting shots and other difficulties associated with his recovery, it was his father who helped him forge a lasting positive attitude toward his disability during the initial fourteen months of chemo treatment, surgery, and then rehab.

We literally became best friends at a quicker pace for father and son I believe. . . . He was very involved. He came to all the meetings, and my mom and dad all throughout the hospital they were the two that were with me . . . for all of the surgery, the chemotherapy sessions. . . . My dad always used to have the tough-skin attitude . . . just tough it up a little bit, you can manage, and be strong and that kind of attitude. But the one thing my dad used to always do, was when I thought I wasn't going to be able to play sports, or be active, or anything for that matter, I had a lot of support from him on almost literally picking me up and going, you know, let's go do this. Hey, you can't ride a bike, let's go get a scooter and try to make this happen. Find ways to work around it, and still manage your life. . . . For me to be active as a one-legged individual, and I honestly think that, my dad's outlook, has kind of made the bigger impact only because when I look at me with my children, and even just before I had my children, when it was me and my fiancée, kind of just young twenty-somethings finding things to do. It was, let's be active.

Landen, with his dad's prodding, cooperatively managed his recovery in the spirit of a father-son partnership. The resilient spirit Landen's father helped nurture is consistent with the amazement pediatric health care professionals often express when describing children's uncanny ability to confront the potentially demoralizing effects of being in poor health.

Now, seventeen years later, Landen believes that a major outcome of his cancer treatment is that he is far less likely to want to take drugs and painkillers for his ailments. He encourages his daughter to adopt a similar perspective for her basic illnesses and asks her to forge ahead with minimal medicine unless she truly needs antibiotics. His motivation to be active also allows him to spend "outdoor time" with his daughter every day on their five acres of land.

In addition to the expression of genes and the challenges of physical ailments, how a boy is raised and supervised by his family and the interactions the child has with peers, coaches, teachers, and others can make a difference. From a practical standpoint, a young boy's diet is influenced by those who buy, prepare, and serve his food. Similarly, a boy's exercise habits, exposure to formal sports, and risk-taking behaviors hinge to no small degree on what his guardians and siblings say and do. Do parents go out of their way to teach their son certain athletic and physical fitness skills? Do they register him for organized athletics and pay admission and equipment fees? Do parents talk in a meaningful way to their kids about nutrition? Do parents conscientiously monitor their children's decisions concerning sunscreen, helmet use, exposure to and use of guns, neighborhood safety, and the like? Not surprisingly, from my sampling of how fathers initially recall their own upbringing and then describe how they treat their kids, children differ greatly in the types of family circumstances they experience— good and bad.

As a boy transitions from childhood to adolescence and then to young adulthood he is bombarded with images and expectations channeled through the media and others he personally knows. Targeting him as a boy, these gendered messages affect what he thinks about his appearance, fitness and health, and all kinds of risky behaviors, including unprotected sex, alcohol and drugs, smoking, and driving fast. The messages contribute to how first the boy, then the young man, defines his body and self-concept. Seeking respect by acting manly is a common thread woven through the messages. Fortunately, in academic circles, and increasingly in the public's eye, the harmful aspects of manly posturing are more widely challenged.[5] But the push for boys to be manly, to be perceived as hard-core, stoic, competitive, nonempathic, and invincible is still very much a part of our culture, especially among youth. Too often, when young men (and women) embrace certain types of traditional messages, they make unhealthy decisions that harm them and others they know—either immediately or in the long run.

A boy or a man's self-image and the way he frames his understanding of the world around him, including his sense of manliness, is often linked to his experiences with health and fitness. Does a boy see himself as Tivon did, as the sickly child burdened with asthma symptoms who misses school days regularly and sees the hospital as his second home? Or does the obese kid internalize the self-loathing that mirrors the shame of always being the last chosen in neighborhood pickup games? On the brighter side, perhaps a boy thinks of himself as a dedicated, fit, and gifted athlete. Terry, a fifty-two-year-old father with experience raising two preteens of his own and three older stepchildren, has always had this view of himself.

> I lived for sports in high school. And I was all-state in three sports and track, cross country, and basketball is what I did like, from I think five years old on. I just was always really active. I rode my bike to school; I was undefeated

for almost four years in the district in running track and cross country. I had the third fastest time in the United States in high school in the two-mile. . . . My whole life I've been real active. I mean I'm fifty-two now, you know, and I'm still sitting here [in] workout clothes after [the] gym, beating myself up because I just, I guess I just can't stop doing it. It's part of my DNA.

Terry reports too that he never had any illnesses as a kid, although his active life and adventuresome personality resulted in numerous hospital visits for stitches and to have broken bones treated. But these trips were not a sign of weakness, as an illness might have been; they were markers of an athletic, risk-taking masculinity.

Although Terry's life shows a remarkable consistency over time, childhood experiences are not destiny. For better or worse, kids' physical conditions can change over time. The child with significant asthma symptoms may grow out of them over time. The healthy child may first experience symptoms of a chronic illness as a teenager or young adult.

No absolute, indelible path links a boy's fitness profile and health consciousness to how he orients to health concerns when he becomes a man. Kids raised in health-conscious families sometimes grow up to consume a junk food diet and get hooked on drugs. So, too, kids raised on fatty junk food who constantly inhale secondhand smoke from sedentary, heavy-drinking parents sometimes commit themselves to a healthy diet and regular exercise while fashioning a life free of drugs, smoking, and alcohol. To their credit, these kids forge life-altering lessons about discipline and self-respect by witnessing and rejecting their parents' unhealthy habits. In turn, they learn to compensate.

Generally speaking, as boys and girls age they tend to assert more autonomy and make lifestyle choices related to health that are independent of direct parental input. Some kids and men (and women) wholeheartedly embrace their parents' values and duplicate their way of life, some selectively reproduce messages and discard others, and some make a conscious effort to distance themselves from their parents' lifestyle choices that affect health outcomes. But whether they accept, selectively pick and choose, or reject outright the messages they received as kids, men are subjected as youth to the forces that define the health matrix. Fortunately, as boys move into and through their adult years some eventually discard or discount the perspectives, practices, and people that compromised their health during their younger years. Unfortunately, others turn their backs on well-meaning, health-conscious parents and end up making poor health choices for themselves and their children. Whatever path men ultimately take, their outlook on life is always somehow connected to their childhood and adolescent experiences. This is true even if men are only superficially aware of health issues as boys.

A number of the fathers included in this book had fathers who did not exercise, drank too much, were addicted to drugs, and ate poorly. The more recent generation of fathers vowed to live better and longer, sometimes with the lingering thought and desire to live a fuller, healthier life in order to witness and be a part of their adult children and grandchildren's lives.

As I've advocated for many years, we need more progressive policies and programs in our schools, public health agencies, places of worship, and other youth-oriented sites to make boys and young men more mindful of their reproductive health and proactive in their approach to self-care.[6] Creating more productive partnerships between parents and public institutions clearly needs to be part of the social agenda in order to enhance how boys and young men, as well as girls and young women, experience the health matrix.[7]

APPROACHING FATHERHOOD

Health stakes are especially high when a man has opportunities to impregnate someone. A man's perception that he can or cannot procreate is part of his health consciousness. More than twenty years ago I began to think deeply about different aspects of what I call *procreative consciousness*—the multiple levels of awareness a man can have about his ability or inability to create human life. These experiences are created as part of a man's active, wide-awake consciousness and then stored in long-term memory as thoughts and feelings for later retrieval. In some respects a man's ties to the health matrix showcased in this book precede any announcement that he is in fact a "father-in-waiting."

In my interviews with dads I didn't routinely ask them about their sexual and reproductive health practices and concerns prior to becoming fathers. However, men's awareness or ignorance of these matters can have health implications for them, their partners, and their children. A man fully aware of his ability to procreate can make conscious prohealth choices to use condoms and to discuss contraception with his partner. Prior to ever being notified that he's going to become a father, the self-reflective man may think about how his job, leisure activities, type of underwear, folic acid deficiency, smoking, drugs, or toxic chemicals he's exposed to in his neighborhood or at work could compromise his sperm. He may worry that poor sperm quality can impede the probability of conception as well as increase the chances that children will be born with birth defects or develop chronic illnesses.[8] Some servicemen have this mind-set when they bank sperm prior to being deployed to combat zones where chemical weapons might be used. Ideally, prior to ever becoming a biological father, a boy or man can consciously make healthy choices to lower the risk for poor health outcomes linked to conception, gestation, childbirth, and future child rearing.

Men's heightened awareness of this sort, though possible, appears to be relatively rare. Unfortunately, most teenage and young adult men do not spend sufficient time thinking about their ability to father children. That half of pregnancies in the United States are unplanned shows that many men are largely oblivious or indifferent to their procreative abilities. Many are simply careless about the sexual risks they take. Presumably, this pattern of ignorance and recklessness can be altered under the right set of circumstances.

Those conditions call for more than what my father said to me as I was growing up—which was absolutely nothing—or the vague messages I offered my eldest son, who typically visited only in the summers. I was impressed with how Joseph handled this issue as a father of three adolescent boys and a girl. In my eyes he's the poster dad for keeping it real when talking with his sons about the world of sex and relationships. He wants to put them in an ideal position to make informed decisions. As he says,

> There's a tradition that I take the boy on his twelfth birthday out to dinner on a dad-and-son date and they get to pick the restaurant and they don't realize why until we get there and I start the conversation. . . . [We are going to go] over everything they ever wanted to know and didn't even want to know especially around the dinner table, about sex and dating and STDs and everything. And, my oldest son was horrified. He picked to go to Chili's and we sat right in the bar area [where] they have the high-top tables and we were really the only two and he's like, Dad, you're not really talking about this. . . . I said we're

going to be here talking until you answer my questions and I feel that you're listening and we go over everything I want to talk about. I said this is going to be a very long and uncomfortable conversation or we can do this pretty quick. And you know, I'd go over a few things and then I'd quiz him on it. Then I'd go over a few things and then I'd quiz him on it. And still to this day, in reference to the genital warts looking like cauliflower . . . he cringes if I'm gonna have cauliflower for dinner.

During the birthday dinner talk, Joseph covers a wide range of topics beyond just sex, STDs, contraception, and pregnancy. He covers homosexuality, prostitution, pornography, masturbation, and more. In doing so, he asks them what they "feel about them . . . is that something that they're interested in or feel like they would like to do or like to try or have tried." Joseph even had several poignant conversations with one of his sons and his girlfriend after Joseph's wife caught the son fondling the girl at the house. To be thorough, he talked to each of them by themselves and then he talked to them as a couple with and without his wife present. Just recently, Joseph also started a conversation with his wife about their eleven-year-old daughter's upcoming transition through puberty; he's not sure though whether he and his wife will jointly talk to the daughter or if the mother will do it by herself.

Although this level of involvement was not the norm, some fathers, though clearly not all, had intimate conversations with their kids. Joseph and I both hope that his talks pay dividends by helping his sons avoid sexually transmitted diseases and unplanned pregnancies.

Unlike Joseph, some fathers face the additional challenge of figuring out how to process the news that one of their adolescent or young adult children is part of the LGBT community. Because young people from earlier eras were less likely to come out than their counterparts today, an increasing number of fathers find themselves navigating this unexpected terrain. One fifty-nine-year-old father, Zeke, had been in the public health field for more than a decade when he learned that his nineteen-year-old son was gay. As a gay man himself, Zeke says that he's been supportive of his son's sexual orientation and has shared some of his firsthand knowledge about life as a gay man with him, even though Zeke downplays how helpful he's been. Because Zeke has extensive professional experience working with HIV issues and has seen most of his previous friends die from AIDS, the value of "protecting oneself from becoming infected" is engrained in his mind. Not surprisingly, Zeke has been very active in having conversations with his son about HIV. Although straight dads can be equally supportive, they are more likely than gay dads to need additional guidance in figuring out how best to support their child. Fortunately, more and more support resources have been made available to parents who accept their LGBT children and are eager to help them.[9]

GETTING BABY NEWS

A father's decision to have or to avoid intimate talks with his child about reproductive health, or any conversation about health, fitness, or well-being, will be colored by his personal and interpersonal histories. Long before a biological father engages his adolescent child, he navigates a fathering path that predates the child's birth. It is here—before a man actually becomes a legal father—that I begin to show how fathers describe their entry into the father-child health matrix.

To initiate men's storytelling as fathers I asked some version of the question: What was it like to learn that you were going to become a father for the first time? When a man is told that he's impregnated someone, he steps into a web of social life that includes his future child, the expectant mother, himself, and sometimes others. A man can focus on what becoming a father will mean for his expectant child, the mother, and his own self-interests, including his health, fitness, and romantic relationship goals.

Sometimes just the news that they are going to become fathers can propel men to adopt healthier choices and forgo their patterns of high-risk choices, including drugs, alcohol, smoking, criminal activity, and motorcycle riding. Fathers can also decide to eat better and exercise more frequently because they are anxious about losing their children's respect and love. Granted, it is tricky to disentangle whether it is raising children or the general maturation process that affects fathers' risk taking and their switch to healthier choices. That said, some men adamantly profess that they intentionally either changed their ways when they learned that they were going to become fathers or that they altered their lifestyle because their children pressured them.[10]

For me, the transition to full-fledged procreative consciousness came in the dead of winter, in the middle of my senior year in high school. I was focused on honing my basketball skills and doing all that I could to ensure that my team made the playoffs. I was highly motivated because a poorly timed bout with mononucleosis had forced me to miss the playoff experience the previous year. Outside of basketball, my cheerleader girlfriend and I were on the cusp of summoning the courage to end a long-term relationship that no longer seemed right for either of us. Fate, however, was not our friend. Before we could redirect our lives on our own terms, we learned that she was five months pregnant. Being naïve teenagers in the mid-1970s, we had, for months, performed mental gymnastics to perpetuate our state of denial, avoiding the rather obvious signs that my girlfriend was nurturing new life. When reality struck, fear, guilt, and shame overwhelmed us. We were confused. Within days, largely guided by our parents' directives, we "chose" marriage to legitimate our involvement in the prenatal process and parenthood. Over the next several months my fears and sentiment of "why me" transformed into anticipation and pride.

Decades later, in a different marriage, and presumably a little wiser, I found myself on the more proactive side of the family planning continuum. In my mind having an extra six months or year to sort out employment and housing issues would have been ideal, but fears that waiting might affect my wife's health trumped those practical considerations. From a health perspective, conceiving a child as soon as possible was the more strategic decision. As my wife and I stared at the over-the-counter pregnancy strip in our bathroom a few months later, my eyes widened and reflected bliss when I saw the blue shading signaling a positive test.

As someone who studies fatherhood for a living and who regularly teaches a course called Sociology of Reproduction and Gender, I was eager to rediscover firsthand the worlds of prenatal classes, obstetrics, and labor and delivery. Unlike my first paternity experience, when I was naïve, overwhelmed, and intimidated by the medical community, I assumed that I would play a more active role in all phases of the pregnancy, labor, delivery, and infant care. Medical staff prevented me from seeing my first son being born—apparently because his mother's final stage of labor had been chemically induced. I was determined to be in the delivery room for my second son's birth, no matter what the circumstances.

Just as I had reacted differently when I learned about the conceptions that culminated in the births of my two sons, other fathers variously describe their initial reactions. Most report being in good spirits when they discovered they were going to be a dad and pass on their genes for the first time. Often with glimmering eyes and a smile, they say things like: "pretty amazing," "wow," "exciting," "thrilled," "ecstatic," "fantastic," and "greatest joy."

A few fathers admit that the news was less than ideal, but they are reluctant to acknowledge openly, retrospectively at least, that they were put off by it. Words like "scared," "uncertain," and "very daunting" were used, but only on a rare occasion did a father characterize it less favorably. Sixteen years ago, news of an unplanned pregnancy threatened the partying lifestyle Gerald cherished before he became a devoted single dad. "I was just more interested in going out to the clubs and you know, meeting women and things like that. So, as bad as it sounds, I just thought maybe a kid would just stop all that and I was like, 'I'm not ready to stop.'" Plenty of fathers are upset when they hear that they are responsible for an unplanned pregnancy, but unlike Gerald, many turn their back and only indirectly affect their child's health by their lack of involvement. Those who walk away are not the type of father I incorporate into this book.

A man who thinks conventionally about men's and women's roles in family and work is more likely than the profeminist man to imagine a simple transition to becoming a future dad, "Wow, I've created my own kid . . . I'm passing on my DNA." Aside from his raw excitement about being a dad, he may only register real concern about his ability to generate the money to raise a baby. In contrast, when a man with progressive beliefs about men's and women's roles in society discovers that he's going to be a father, he may entertain a more complex set of concerns. Alongside the immediate "wow" feelings, a man with progressive views about gender may ponder his responsibilities for taking care of a child's daily needs from infancy to adulthood. Thus the breaking news about a future baby may prompt him to figure out not just the financial side of fathering but how he and perhaps his partner are going to adjust work, family, and leisure schedules to care for a child. Although specific health issues are unlikely to dominate a father's mind-set at this point, those with a family history of genetic disorders or whose partners have such a family history may be more apt to weave concerns about health into their thinking.

Whatever a man's belief system, he will learn about his future paternity as part of a larger social context that will affect the extent to which he sees himself as being ready to be a good father. Is he in a stable relationship with the right partner? Has he on his own or with his partner sufficiently realized his young adult dreams for play, travel, and adventure? Is he financially set to provide for a child in a manner he deems worthy? Are his home and neighborhood conducive to raising a child? Is he emotionally mature enough to care for a baby and child? These and other circumstances will either constrain or foster how he navigates the health matrix during the pregnancy and beyond.

EMBRACING THE PRENATAL WORLD

By now, most of us have seen one of the many depictions or representations of a pregnant man in popular films, science fiction, performance art, and even real life. One of the better known examples appeared more than twenty years ago, in the American comedy *Junior*, when Arnold Schwarzenegger played a scientist who underwent a male pregnancy to verify the viability of a fertility drug he had invented. An episode in the *Star Trek: Enterprise* series, "Unexpected," featured a male human who was pregnant with the offspring of a female of another species. About fifteen years ago, performance artists Virgil Wong and Lee Mingwei produced an elaborate hoax website *POP! The First Male Pregnancy* that showcased various aspects of Mr. Mingwei's fictitious pregnancy.[11] And then there is Thomas Beatie, a transgender man who had, as of November 2012, given birth to a girl and two boys, with the first child having been born in 2008. Media coverage of this case was fairly extensive. Barbara Walters talked about Mr. Beatie's second pregnancy on *The View* and Anderson Cooper interviewed Mr. Beatie on CNN about his legal battles to have his marriage recognized and his divorce from the coparent finalized. The Guinness World Records even acknowledged Mr. Beatie as the world's "first married man to give birth."[12]

Most recently, a new fad that uses the "labor pain contraction simulator" has penetrated pop culture. Men are volunteering to have patches placed on their abdomens that generate electrical currents, creating intense contractions. Various You Tube videos now show men subjecting themselves to these simulations in order to get a small taste of what a woman experiences during labor.[13]

Although my interviews are not as titillating as Hollywood depictions, science fiction, or transgender female-to-male accounts of men gestating fetuses, my interviews do show how men in a diverse sample over the past few decades have found ways to be involved in different aspects of the prenatal process. The pregnancies the men describe cover a wide range of circumstances: some were meticulously planned, others unwelcome surprises; some occurred in long-term marriages, others in casual friendships; some happened quickly and naturally, others after years of trying, sometimes with the help of a fertility specialist; some involved straight couples; others included gay men donating sperm or being linked to a pregnancy that led to a baby's adoption; some were uncomplicated pregnancies, others became high-risk events—ending with either a healthy baby, a child with special needs, or an infant's death. During the pregnancy, and sometimes even prior to conception, many men felt they had entered into a serious coparental partnership that deserved their time and energy.

How do men describe their involvement in their partner's pregnancy, and what might be the implications of their actions for the health of the mother and baby? Generally speaking, research shows that when a pregnant woman's partner is more active and supportive during the pregnancy, the woman takes better care of herself and the baby is healthier.[14] During a pregnancy, a man can do all sorts of things to express his commitment either to his partner, the baby, or both.[15] A man's specific motivation is not always apparent, however.

When I learned that my wife was pregnant with Phoenix, I went to all of her doctor's visits. Although my flexible work schedule made this relatively easy, I would like to think I would have figured out a way to go even if my schedule had been more rigid. It seems now, as it did then, to be a no-brainer that a man in my position should support his partner while being attentive to the health of the child he helped to create. Fortunately, I'm not alone in how I think about these matters. Several dads proudly asserted that they attended every appointment their partner had with an ob-gyn or midwife.[16] Many went to most appointments, and almost everyone recalled going to at least some of the consultations. Like me, they were content with how they were treated by medical staff. They felt they had been sufficiently acknowledged and incorporated into the flow of the discussion, and that their questions were answered to their satisfaction.

A significant majority also enrolled with their partner in at least one prenatal course. My wife and I made the rounds to a general birthing class and a series of prenatal classes, including a breast-feeding workshop and a class on buying and using a baby seat. As I recall, the pregnant women asked more questions than their partners, but most of the men seemed reasonably comfortable and were attentive.

Still, as my interviews confirm, some men feel out of place in what they see as a woman's domain. Jared, an African American high school dropout with rural southern roots, was twenty-nine in 2003 when he became a dad. How did he feel about going to a prenatal class with his girlfriend? "Just weird, man. I was like the only guy in there, you know, just trying to help out. I went to one class, man, and I just said it's too many women in there, man, I don't want to be in there with a bunch of women. I'm real old school, so, like, if I'm around a bunch of women and I'm the only guy, I kind of feel kind of weirded out. . . . I was just raised like that." Troy, a white man who also had a rural southern upbringing, confides that when he was twenty-five in the early 1990s and had his first daughter he went to a Lamaze class with his wife. Like Jared, he "felt a little out of place." Troy explains, "because I was raised as husband and wife, dad as the head of the household and does all of the hard work, and mom handles all of that stuff [pregnancy, child-birth, child care], I was feeling a little strange at first, not really uncomfort-able just odd 'cause a lot of the women were there without their spouse, no husband, a lot of unwed mothers."

Stories like Jared's and Troy's shout out for attention. Health educators need to do a better job of making their programs attractive to men from all sorts of cultural backgrounds. Clearly, the biggest challenge is to entice men with traditional views about men and women to come to appreciate the value of learning more about the role they can play in promoting their partner's and their child's health beyond making money and paying doc-tors' bills.

Collectively, the men shared other ways they got involved informally with the pregnancy—directly or indirectly. Many men described how they talked, sang, played music, or "beat box rapped" to their baby in utero. Landen, the father who had lost his leg to cancer as a teenager, wrote and played original songs for both of his kids when his wife was pregnant. After we ended the formal portion of our Skype interview, I persuaded Landen to perform one of his touching songs. A few men, presumably without Landen's talents, smiled broadly as they shared stories about how they placed headphones on their partner's belly and played music.

At least two of the younger first-time dads downloaded specialized computer apps like Baby Bump to their phone. Barry, a twenty-eight-year-old father of a four-month-old, used this app almost daily during his wife's pregnancy and recommended it to others. The app allowed Barry to retrieve information about standard fetal developmental that he synchronized to his own child's prenatal age. These programs, I suspect, will grow in popularity as tech-savvy men find new ways to express themselves as competent, nurturing dads.

Some men incorporated people other than their partner into their prenatal experience. Joseph reported that he and his wife met with five other pregnant couples over a period of months to read and discuss a book about pregnancy expectations. Meanwhile, Landen shared fond memories of going to a "Daddy and Me" workshop while Nick chatted with his work colleagues and successfully secured the recommendation for a well-respected midwife.

One of the major innovations in reproductive technology during the twentieth century was the introduction of the pregnancy ultrasound, which offers future parents, medical staff, and others the opportunity to see an image of a developing fetus. This remarkable development gives men their first chance to establish a visually based attachment to a yet-to-be-born living form they helped produce.[17] After talking to eighteen British men multiple times during their partner's pregnancy and after their child's birth, Jan Draper concludes that the visual element of an ultrasound carries special significance for men in making the pregnancy real.

In 1976 I never got to see a prenatal image of my eldest son. Fast forward to 2007 and I not only saw real-time ultrasound images of Phoenix, I was also treated to a 4D video version that brought him to life in a magnificent way. I replayed his 4D performance on my computer, and his ultrasound image found a prominent place on the refrigerator door next to other family photos. I even incorporated the image into my PowerPoint lecture on procreative identity and fathering.

As they were for me, the ultrasound moments were significant experiences for many of the fathers. Seeing a prenatal image of one's child was a transformative experience for a few men because it helped to crystallize their identity as a father. Warren, age twenty-two but already the father of three preschool children, interpreted the first ultrasound he saw as the "actualization" moment that allowed him to realize that a child that was partly "his" was living inside his partner. One father was so thrilled with his first child's ultrasound that he laminated it. A father of four young children described the first ultrasound as "magic." The 4D ultrasound was "unforgettable," says a twenty-seven-year-old Puerto Rican father with a new baby just twelve days old. I tend to agree.

But surprisingly, and unlike my own experience, several men were not impressed with the ultrasounds for their babies. Jonathan, a physician, talks casually about how his medical training shaped his processing of his first child's ultrasound. Although he didn't let on to his wife, he was in "diagnostic mode." His mind raced, as he wondered "how much amniotic fluid there was and was there a beating heart and what was the hip-to-trunk ratio and I was too much thinking medically to make sure that he was healthy, as opposed to [thinking] wow, 'there's my kid on the sonogram.'" Jonathan admits to having at most a "small connection" to the fetus because having his "doctor's hat on" limited his ability to relate to the fetus as a nonmedical father might.

I sensed too that a few dads' muted reactions resulted from their unrealistic expectations about the fetal image an ultrasound produces. A couple of men were even disoriented when they tried to figure out their child's shape from images that captured early fetal development.

Fetal images are now engrained in popular culture and ultrasounds are standard practice in Western obstetrics.[18] We see the images in advertisements as well as in campaign material for the pro-life movement.[19] Parents and others talk about them routinely. It should be no surprise that the cultural landscape compels some prospective fathers to be underwhelmed or disappointed by the images they eventually see.

Ultrasound technology and the sophisticated prenatal testing currently available expand the options for how a man experiences the health matrix during the prenatal period.[20] Today, parents-to-be can rely on ultrasound or biochemical/genetic screening to determine more easily if their child has particular genetic disorders. The man can weigh in on whether he even wants a certain test performed. And if the test identifies abnormalities, he can share his views on what, if anything, should be done to terminate a pregnancy or make preparations for who will care for the child and how the care will be arranged.

A prospective father is not limited to making a difference for his pregnant partner and unborn child through his involvement in prenatal visits and participating in prenatal courses. He can try to contribute in various ways, but it may be difficult at times to distinguish whether the father is saying or doing something to target his child, the mother, or both. For example, several men talk about encouraging their partners to quit smoking during pregnancy. A mother and child both stand to benefit when this advice is heeded.

Some men found themselves unexpectedly caring for women who had high-risk pregnancies. By his own account, once Delmore learned that the mother might lose the pregnancy, he "made her quit her job." He says, "I just had to man up, just make sure everything was gonna be okay." In the end, he had a baby girl who is now nine and, aside from her mild case of asthma, has been healthy. The mother of Dustin's child had gestational diabetes and threw up every day. She struggled with epilepsy and sometimes had two seizures a day because she couldn't keep her medicine down. She was hospitalized a lot, an entire week on one occasion, because she was so dehydrated. Dustin describes himself as doing all of the work around the house, including caring for his older daughter and two stepchildren while also holding down a paid job. He tried to help her as much as he could. Ultimately, the baby boy was born three months prematurely, remained in the ICU for a week, and was in the hospital for a month before being released to go home. Like Delmore's girl, the boy had asthma but has grown out of it for the most part. There's no way to say with certainty how much of a difference Delmore or Dustin made in these pregnancies. It seems reasonable to assume, though, that the support these men gave their partners contributed to better health outcomes for the mother and child.

What a father does can sometimes indirectly affect the health of the baby and mother. Emotionally, a man can support his pregnant partner in various ways. With the pregnancy fresh in his mind for his twelve-day-old son, I asked Diego to elaborate on why he thought the sessions were "exciting" and why he loved to go with his partner to visit the midwife at the birthing center. "My wife would express things to the midwife that she didn't express to me. So I would always learn new things about how my wife was feeling, about the pregnancy." Diego's wife talked a lot about her fears, especially how the baby might hold her back from pursuing her own goals like traveling outside the country to teach. Hearing his wife share such fears with the midwife helped Diego get a better handle on what his wife was experiencing and gave him an opportunity to encourage her and ease her stress.

Unlike Diego, who was involved in a planned pregnancy in a committed marriage, many men, like Gerald at age twenty-five, learn they have a baby on the way outside a serious relationship. In Gerald's case, the mother-to-be was only twenty. With a sheepish grin, Gerald explains, "I was into women. So, she was maybe like one of a few." Reflecting on the sentiments he had after the initial shock wore off, he continues, "I looked at her different . . . she's gonna be the mother of my child . . . I looked at her with a lot more respect, a lot more um affection . . . I cared about her well-being . . . to make sure she was healthy, in her pregnancy." He recalls that they "probably became like boyfriend and girlfriend maybe for about eight months" but separated before his child was born. Circumstances like these typically result in the father being less involved in caregiving activities for the mother and child. Prior to the separation, Gerald claims he was "always" bringing the mother food, water, apple juice, and whatever she needed. He would often go and just hang out with his girlfriend because her mother worked. Gerald claims he never went to any of the doctor's appointments because he wasn't informed about them until afterward, or his girlfriend's mother went instead.

Gerald's reality illustrates how others, like a mother wanting to protect her young daughter and eager to be a grandma, can slip into the health matrix at an early stage and potentially alter a man's experience by usurping his role. People's actions can produce positive, negative, or mixed results for how the father relates to his child's health needs in the short- and long-term.

The dads I spoke with routinely mention being on board with breast-feeding before the child's birth and encourage it. Whether their partners would confirm this I cannot say. However, it does appear that most of the dads embrace the public health campaign message that breast-feeding has distinct health advantages for the child, such as protecting a child from illnesses and from developing allergies.[21] Researchers and lactation consultants who focus on breast-feeding practices offer additional perspectives on how parents navigate and feel about breast-feeding.[22] One view is that even though some fathers encourage it in principle prior to a child's birth, their sentiments shift once breast-feeding becomes a many-times-a-day reality. They feel that breast-feeding interferes with their chances to bond with their child. Some also feel the baby disrupts their relationship with their mate.[23] No one can say with certainty how widespread this pattern is, but I suspect some men feel this way. Yet if lactating mothers are willing and able to use a breast pump to extract milk, fathers can simulate nursing by bottle feeding their children breast milk.

When Phoenix was a newborn I loved the intimate moments I shared with him using my wife's expressed milk, which we packaged and froze. I was thrilled to be fully in charge of his feedings for a three-day period when my wife left home on a business trip. Unfortunately, my feeding opportunities faded because within several months Phoenix started to reject taking milk from a bottle. A few of the fathers shared similar sentiments about how a breast pump gave them snippets of intimacy with their baby.

Another point the breast-feeding experts raise involves what Phyllis Rippeyoung and Mary Noonan call the "dark side" of breast-feeding— how this practice sometimes reinforces a traditional and unequal division of child care that constrains mothers.[24] The argument goes that when a mom breast-feeds, heterosexual parents slide into domestic and paid work patterns that lead to the mother doing most or all of the hands-on baby care. The mom is then more readily viewed as the primary caregiver and the dad becomes the helper and babysitter. Because bottle feeding—one of the more enjoyable forms of child care—is unavailable, the father is less inclined to be active in changing diapers or tending to a colicky baby.

Others interpret the interpersonal dynamics of breast-feeding differently. They suggest that instead of perpetuating traditional child care patterns, breast-feeding can prompt a nurturing, attentive father to get more involved with other child care and baby hygiene activities because he is unable to be in charge of feeding sessions.

What does the available research on parents and breast-feeding from the United States tell us? Rippeyoung and Noonan used the Early Childhood Longitudinal Study (Birth Cohort)—a large-scale study of families that included 10,688 babies born in 2001—to compare survey responses of fathers of nine-month-old children in two types of families based on the children's degree of exposure to breast-feeding.[25] Looking at eleven different measures of father involvement, including such things as changing diapers, washing and bathing, putting to sleep, soothing, attending doctors' visits, and staying at home with a sick child, they found that dads of breast-fed babies report doing less than dads whose children are not being breast-fed. But when the researchers gathered reports at the two-year mark, no differences appeared between fathers of infants who were never breast-fed and those who were breast-fed for less than six months.

I agree with the authors' inclination to reject what they label the "optimistic advocate" position that would resign us to feeling good that the pattern doesn't persist long-term. Nor should we adopt the "formula-feeding feminist" interpretation and discourage mothers from breast-feeding just because there's an empirical pattern of infant care among breast-feeding parents that reflects a form of gender inequality. Rather we need to highlight the findings about breast-feeding and father involvement and assume a "feminist advocate" position. To do so, we must encourage public health campaigns promoting breast-feeding to focus more attention on what a father can and should do to be a more profeminist and active participant in infant care.

My own experience over several decades runs contrary to the recently documented general patterns. Back in the 1970s Scott was formula-fed from the start, and while I did some bottle feeding, I regrettably did little else in terms of infant care beyond being a playmate. I surely did very little, if any, diaper changing. In stark contrast, I was highly engaged thirty-plus years later in every aspect of Phoenix's infant and toddler care despite Phoenix being a breast-fed kid for roughly thirty months. Oddly, I took great pleasure in changing Phoenix's diaper and never turned down the opportunity. It was not a chore or simply an exercise in hygiene maintenance for me—it was one of our special bonding rituals. I prided myself on figuring out tricks to increase my speed and avoid any unnecessary mess while keeping him content even in the most confined settings like airplane bathrooms. My life experience demonstrates that men can be motivated to transition away from a traditional, gender-typed approach to child care to a much more profeminist practice. Getting traditionally oriented men to make this shift prior to their first child being born is obviously the ideal.

A national study by Rippeyoung and Noonan of 1,313 women who gave birth to their first child between 1980 and 1993[26] further complicates the message that "breastfeeding is best."[27] Women who breast-feed tend to be white, college educated, and married, and this is often for economic reasons,. The study finds that long-duration breast-feeding (six months or more) leads to women spending less time in the labor market, thereby reducing both their short- and long-term earnings. According to the authors, "encouraging a mother to breastfeed at the cost of lowering the family's income may not be the best way toward better health for mother and child." Although fathers sometimes clean breast pump equipment, fetch the baby from the crib late at night to bring to the mother, or even do extra housework to free up a little time for the mother, it's not clear if dads do or say anything to manage the possible hidden financial costs that accompany breast-feeding, especially for women who breast-feed for six months or longer.

Because I had my sons thirty-one years apart—in 1976 and 2007—I've formed my own impressions of how the hospital-based birthing model has evolved to integrate fathers more fully into that magnificent moment of labor and delivery. When I was excluded from Scott's delivery, I dropped my sleep-deprived body to the linoleum hallway floor and tried to rest while I awaited the doctor's eventual announcement that my son had been born and everything was all right with mother and child. I was too tired and too young to challenge the doctor's decision to exclude me from the birth. I was present throughout the twenty-six hours of grueling labor that momentarily snatched sanity from the mother's mind. All things considered, I think I did reasonably well trying to be a nurturing partner. But I also sensed then, and recognize much better now, that I was not the best medical advocate for my son's mother during the labor process. Being a young eighteen, I was intimidated by the medical model and felt uncomfortable challenging anyone or critically assessing any procedure. Had Scott's mother insisted that I go with her to the delivery room I'm sure I would have been more assertive, although I would have been reluctant to challenge vigorously the doctor's authority and "wisdom."

That shyness changed by the time Phoenix was getting ready to enter the outside world. In the labor room, I discussed at length with one of the nurses why it is not patient-friendly to have the monitor assessing the baby's vital signs situated in a manner that made it difficult for my wife to observe. My comments were anchored in the feminist readings I use in the classroom that challenge the routines, assumptions, and communication style associated with the medical model of hospital-based birthing. The conventional view downplays or ignores women's experiential understanding of their pregnant bodies and limits their autonomy.[28] I never thought to have that sort of discussion with medical staff when Scott was born.

When Phoenix was born, I was next to my wife in the delivery room and witnessed his first breaths and sounds. I hovered over him as he was wiped off, weighed and measured, examined, and swaddled. The following day my personal request to be present to hold his hand during his circumcision was honored. I never thought to ask this question with my first son and I doubt whether I would have been accommodated if I had.

I discovered firsthand that much has changed in how hospital personnel treat prospective fathers during labor and delivery. Unfortunately, I can only speculate on how being a teenager versus being a middle-aged man may have altered the different medical professionals' reactions to me and my perceptions of them at the time as well as now. I do know that, contrary to my first fathering experience, I had met and talked with the obstetrician many times prior to her delivering my son. She knew and seemingly respected me, and I trusted her. I was also a more knowledgeable and assertive advocate for my wife and child the second time.

Make no mistake about it though: childbirth rituals have been transformed in the United States. Judith Walzer Leavitt, a medical historian and women's studies professor, creatively uses brief diaries, interviews, birth stories, and public documents produced largely by middle-class white parents to establish how successive cohorts of fathers and mothers from the 1940s to the 1980s transitioned from seeing men's participation in their baby's birth as an afterthought to a possibility, to a privilege, to a right.[29] Her analysis of popular culture—cartoons, TV sitcoms, popular press magazine articles, and newspaper commentaries—also shows how the change was set in motion. My interviews with fathers provide a more contemporary reminder that the vast majority of fathers during the past two decades have become more attentive to health issues for their pregnant partners and children, and they take it for granted that they are going to be present during that momentous occasion of their child's birth.

3 ⇥ ROUTINES, RITUALS, AND CARE

JEREMY, A LEADING VEGAN activist with a similarly minded wife, glows when talking about the wonderful relationship he has with his wife and their close connection with Sarah, their only child. He feels especially lucky to have a tranquil, life-affirming relationship with his teenage daughter.

Sarah, a cross-country runner, frequently does training runs with her forty-four-year-old dad, who "enjoys spending time with her running" at practices or on their own. Because Sarah has no interest in driving despite being seventeen, Jeremy regularly takes her to practice and then sometimes runs with her and her teammates. But Jeremy is much more than a running buddy for Sarah. He has become Sarah's informal trainer: he diligently studies workout and nutritional regimens, and Sarah trusts his judgment. For several years he's shared advice with her about training routines and diet. Their partnership is unique.

Since becoming parents, Jeremy and his wife have shared lots of family time with their daughter doing physical activities like hiking and biking.

The parents have also talked to her frequently about the nutritional value of the meals they prepare for her. Jeremy is keenly aware of these conversations because his diet is outside the mainstream. He wants to avoid the potential "slam on being vegan" that he believes others direct toward those vegans who are sick a lot. Speaking about himself and his wife, Jeremy claims that "we've been much more aware of nutrition, and, health issues, because we're vegan, . . . [unlike] the average parent." In addition, Jeremy's professional responsibilities working for an organization that promotes a vegan lifestyle keep him informed about health-related matters, information that he shares with his daughter.

The bliss Jeremy has experienced as a father for the last sixteen years stands in stark contrast to the stress and exhaustion he encountered during his first year of fatherhood. In telling his life story about fathering, he intentionally distinguishes between the first year, when Sarah could not "communicate and get around," and all the other years. "She cried a lot. She slept very irregularly. We [wife and Jeremy] spent many nights walking the halls of the apartment building with her in a sling and trying to just keep her from screaming, driving her in the car, to try to get her to fall asleep, so, the first year, was really an endurance test, without any sleep, with this very unhappy child." The stress was so bad during the first year that he began to experience his initial symptoms of a condition that eventually was diagnosed as Crohn's disease—an inflammatory bowel condition. He resists claiming that a "screaming baby" caused his disease but he is quick to note the peculiar timing of events.

Whether it was during that horrendous first year or any of the more pleasurable ones since, Jeremy has committed himself to getting into a daily rhythm of spending time with and caring for his daughter. Jeremy is a devoted, nurturing dad who is concerned about his daughter's overall well-being. Even before Sarah was born, Jeremy joined his wife at meetings with a midwife. He favored breast-feeding and assumed that his wife would breast-feed, but he was unable to recall having a formal discussion with her about it.[1] Because Sarah had a fairly typical pregnancy, with morning sickness through the first three months and no complications, there wasn't much that Jeremy could do to affect his unborn child's health.

With reproductive physiology being what it is, a man—even an attentive father like Jeremy—has at best only a few indirect options to affect his child's health during the prenatal months. However, things change dramatically once a child is born and is no longer by necessity tied to the mother's gestational gifts of life. A dad is free to focus on the child's health in numerous ways. The specific options vary, of course, as the child's developmental needs change over time. Jeremy transitioned from the draining nightly rituals of walking his colicky infant to sleep to the invigorating running dates that challenge him to keep pace with his very fit daughter.

In many respects the most effective health-conscious dad is a proactive one. He is able to anticipate his child's needs and respond to them effectively. Broadly speaking, a dad can do things with and for his child directly by taking care of general hygiene needs, administering medications, encouraging a particular diet or type of exercise, and being attentive to various safety needs.

Indirectly, he can leave an imprint by gathering health-related information from different sources to inform a decision about his child. For example, a father might speak to behavioral experts in autism prior to experimenting with or rejecting drug therapy for his autistic child. A father can advocate for or against his healthy child's need for a flu vaccination as he explores options and lobbies for a particular course of action by talking to medical professionals and negotiating with a potentially reluctant coparent. And a father can also model healthy choices by what he does for himself: committing to a nutritious diet, exercising regularly, arranging timely doctor visits, and establishing a thoughtful spiritual practice.

BEING ENGAGED DIRECTLY

What a father does for his child and for himself within the health matrix can often be labeled a routine or ritual. Typically, a routine is thought to be some sort of regular procedure or habitual activity. A ritual is created when a symbolic element is added to a set of acts or routines that are regularly repeated. When performed in the context of family life, a ritual can provide members with a sense of identity and belonging. It often leads to powerful emotions and reminiscing among family members.

This is certainly true for how running has become a staple in the life of Jeremy's family. Jeremy began to take running more seriously because his wife was an avid runner and her siblings were runners too. Sarah followed her parents' lead and took up running competitively in middle school. So for several years they have nurtured their identity as a happy, running family. Jeremy even does the timing and his wife keeps the scores for Sarah's home meets.

Running has also been a unifying force in the family life of Troy, a forty-five-year-old military officer and father to three daughters. But in Troy's world, it was his sixteen-year-old daughter who inspired him to put more time and effort into getting fit. Troy began to run with his daughter when she got involved with track in middle school. He ran up to forty-five miles a week with his daughter in the summer. Although Troy jokingly describes his six-foot five-inch and once 240-pound frame as more suitable for pulling a plow, he takes considerable pride in setting an example in perseverance for his three daughters. So too, his commitment to running inspired his wife to become a serious runner.

Training for and doing obstacle course races together with his children has been a great experience for Giovanni, a fifty-year-old endurance athlete with five kids ages ten to twenty-two. He describes how he and his children sometimes have difficulty "expressing ourselves and our thoughts and our feelings" and characterizes exercising together as a "bonding" experience. For Giovanni, it provides an alternative way to interact with his kids that balances out those occasions where he needs to be a parent and "lay down the law." So he sees it as "really fun to be able to do stuff with them and share interests together . . .'cause it leads to deeper conversations and more sharing of heart on heart versus just doing stuff together."

Some of my own bike rides with Phoenix foster those intimate moments of sharing when he reflects out loud about his friends, hopes and dreams, things that are bothering him, and life in general. In fact, it was on one of our autumn bike rides when Phoenix was a first-grader that he broached the subject of having his first "girlfriend." On subsequent rides we talked about what this experience meant to him. As we both grew more comfortable with his biking prowess I was able to spend less time monitoring his cycling habits and more time chatting about our lives.

Our most powerful mountain-biking rituals emerged once we began to explore a few local nature trails. It was a magical moment when we saw a deer close up five minutes into our first ride on the paved Hawthorne trail. A few weeks later, we spotted forty deer during a six-hour excursion on the challenging off-road trails of San Felasco State Park. The joy of that day cemented our desire to use our bikes to both exercise and journey through nature. It was then too that we adopted the practice of comparing the number of deer we see with the number of fellow riders we encounter on a given ride. Our deer-spotting rituals have made it easier for me to pass on to Phoenix the affinity for nature that Richard Louv wrote about so passionately.[2] The opportunity to take and store photos of wildlife with a smart phone has solidified the meaning of our trail riding rituals for each of us.

Unfortunately, mountain biking had not gained mainstream status when my first son was in elementary school. I believe I was largely oblivious to its existence, and even if I had been one of the earlier adopters, my poor finances would have restricted my options to purchase the necessary equipment. Since the late 1970s and early 1980s, the refinement of mountain-bike technology, the growth of the sport, and community investment in developing trails and parks has meant that more fathers like me have fresh and exciting opportunities to bond with their children through a combination of adventure and fitness activities in nature. Mountain biking extends the lessons associated with the hiking and camping trips fathers have traditionally shared with their children.

Ironically, once I decided, three weeks prior to Phoenix's seventh birthday, to honor his year-long request to get a road bike, our riding time together took a new turn. Over the first two years much of our road riding has taken on more of a "training ride" feel as I prepare him for his competitive youth triathlon races. To compete at a high level he needs to have the right equipment and pay attention to numerous details about efficient cycling and fast transitions onto and off of the bike. These rides, and the transition training, have been less about riding in nature and having casual, intimate conversations, which is part of our mountain-bike experience, and more about my being a coach and motivator—an experience that has led to a fresh type of bonding time as well as friction when I apply too much performance pressure. While finding a comfortable balance between productive motivation and excess pressure is a challenge for coaches in general, it is especially tricky when dealing with one's own child.

I vividly recall our first taste of competitive cooperation on road bikes, which occurred a few days after he started to ride his new bike. About six miles into our ride I challenged him to pick up his pace so that we could prevent another cyclist from overtaking us. Roughly twenty seconds after we began to retrace our path at the turnaround point on the paved bike trail, I noticed a serious cyclist approaching us from the front. I assumed he too would do the turnaround and be on our wheels shortly. When he passed us initially going the other direction, I looked at Phoenix on my right and challenged him by saying, "Let's stay away and not let that guy catch us. He's gonna turn around like we did." With a little prodding, I convinced Phoenix, and we both accelerated. Twenty seconds later I turned around and spotted the rider and warned Phoenix that he was coming. For the next three miles Phoenix and I monitored the trailing rider. At one point Phoenix insisted he had "no more power," so I revised my challenge and told him that we should at least "hold the guy off until we reach Parker Road"—about a mile away. After that "carrot" eventually gave way to his exhausted legs, lungs, and mental focus, I told him to "take my wheel" and draft behind me, which he did. He had watched enough coverage of the Tour de France to understand the basic logic of breakaways and pursuits where riders either leave the peloton (the main group of riders) or try to catch those who have accelerated and gone out ahead of their competitors. We made it to Parker Road in the lead, barely, before being overtaken by a fit-looking man, probably in his early twenties. Our first stab at "team riding" tested Phoenix's limits and gave us a cool workout memory. I've created other occasions since when I've challenged him to go fast and hard as my "teammate."

I waited for over a year for the magical moment when he initiated the ritual and volunteered to push through the fatigue and discomfort. It came on the morning of August 29, 2105, when an athletic-looking man on a road bike passed me and then Phoenix, who was in front setting our pace. We were already going reasonably fast, but the rider established a sizable lead within a minute or so, and then I noticed Phoenix drop down on his handlebars into an aero position and begin to pick up the pace. I followed silently close behind, waiting to see what would unfold with Phoenix's chase. Slowly but decisively, Phoenix reduced the gap over the next two and a half miles and was on the verge of passing the rider when the rider stopped suddenly at a crossroad to check traffic and to make a left turn. Although Phoenix didn't get to feel the mental rush of executing a payback pass on an athletic adult, we shared in the excitement that he had done something new and special.

When fathers spoke to me about their involvement in promoting their kids' health, fitness, and well-being they too often flagged experiences tied to routines and rituals. Sometimes activities emerge organically without much conscious forethought or preparation. Other times, a father deliberately tries to establish a predictable pattern that is meant to bring health and fitness benefits to his child and possibly to himself as well.

Reflecting on their childhoods and their time with their own kids, fathers talked a lot about aspects of gardening, food shopping, meal prep-aration and dinner time, and various forms of physical activity, including sports. Many of these stories bring to life recent research and public debates on childhood obesity and fitness.

Since childhood, I've been a fan of creating rituals with family and friends, and I tend to be a creature of habit in how I approach diet and fit-ness. It feels natural to devise fun rituals to strengthen my bond with Phoe-nix as I try to inspire him to value a healthy lifestyle. When he was a toddler I would sit with him in the afternoon on the preschool porch after picking him up for the day. With his lunchbox in my lap I encouraged him to fin-ish what I had packed for him before we ventured to a neighborhood play-ground. Usually we worked on carrots, grapes, a banana, or a sandwich. Notably, we had purchased those items during one of our grocery store adventures we enjoyed three times a week in which I rolled him around in a carlike cart that we affectionately call the "big green machine." During those excursions I began to introduce him to the world of nutrition and healthy eating based on my commitment to a pescetarian diet, which includes dairy and fish but no meat.

Over the years Phoenix has become my walking companion at the store and has evolved into an eager and meticulous inspector of fruits and veg-etables. By the time he turned six and a half, I estimate that he and I had visited a grocery store well over five hundred times together. Phoenix prides himself on locating flawless tomatoes, red peppers, and corn on the cob. At five, he learned to read nutrition labels and is quite adept at spotting levels of saturated fat, sugar, sodium, protein, and several vitamins. He now even challenges some of my purchases after inspecting a label. And he has, on his own, lectured his mother about her choice of drinking Coke in the house—taking a half-filled bottle from her on one occasion and putting it with the recycle items. I still struggle to get him to eat as many vegetables as I would prefer, but our educational trips to the grocery store have begun to pay divi-dends. Our next step, and a first for me, will be to experiment with planting a vegetable garden.

Gardening

Listening to fathers talk about health issues has emboldened me to consider gardening in order to produce my own family food. I was struck by how many men had distinct childhood memories of tending to family gardens and how many have created gardening experiences with their own kids.

Ramsey, a multiracial twenty-two-year-old with a five-year-old daughter, was raised in rural north central Florida along with his four brothers by a single mom because his father was in prison for most of Ramsey's life. He recalls how he did all the strenuous garden work, getting the soil ready for his mom and then spending an hour or so a day watering, fertilizing, and weeding. Ramsey appreciated his mom's integrating him into the seed selection process by asking what he wanted to plant. "I like greens and stuff like that [so] we planted some kale, some collard greens, some mustard greens, rutabagas, carrots, broccoli—which my daughter she loved it, just going over to the house and pick it right off the plant and eat it."

Ramsey currently lives with his grandmother, and he put in a garden for her six weeks before our interview. Gardening, in his eyes, is "good" and consistent with his current life philosophy. "It saves time; it's healthy things growing straight out the garden. I'm trying to eat healthy, trying to stay in shape and stuff like that. And it's definitely beneficial for me and my grandma."

Ramsey clarifies that the joy he associates with his grandma's garden extends beyond the practical benefits because it brings him closer to his daughter. "Whenever I'm working in the garden I have her out there. She is a vegetarian . . . and so she loves vegetables, every kind. So, she loves watering the garden. She loves the plants, and seeing the bugs. So, it's really cool." He adds, "It's definitely bonding for me and her. It's something that we can do that draws us together."

Brent, a white middle-aged father living in Pennsylvania, also shares fond memories of how gardening had been a great opportunity for him to connect with his kids, who are now in their early twenties. As a child he had been raised in a stable, two-parent family in Maryland with a devoted father who spent lots of ritual time exercising with him. When Brent established his own family, he was blessed with owning plenty of land and talks about how he and his wife incorporated gardening into his interactions with his kids over the years:

It was a very big part of it; we grew a [big] garden every year. It was part of their homeschooling, it was part of our bonding, it was part of our activities. They would help with plowing, tilling, seeding, weeding, harvesting, we would always give them a little section of the garden that was theirs, they could plant whatever they wanted and James would always choose one of the hottest, spiciest peppers I can find, and he would do research, oh wow, if you put lime on it, it makes it hotter, and you know, it got very active. James to this day grows a garden where he's living now. . . . It's actually become a very big part of his life, he loves to garden.

Ramsey and Brent were raised in very different types of households and are currently in different phases of their lives. Yet they both enthusiastically embrace the spirit of gardening and value the process of passing down the tradition from one generation to the next. In the end, whether gardening is born out of financial necessity, a desire to be connected to the land and eat organically, or an opportunity to provide practical homeschooling lessons, dads can use gardening to bond with and educate their children as part of the health matrix. If done well, it may even become part of a family legacy.

One rendition of a family legacy rooted in rural southern living was offered by Wyatt, a fifty-one-year-old African American, who shared his sentiments about his childhood. His description of his typical Sunday afternoon meal reveals a lifestyle tied to the land that is largely beyond my immediate personal experience, and one that is foreign to most American kids and families today.

Okras come out of the garden, we ate them. Corn, we ate corns on the cob, my mom would grill them and that was less food she had to buy out the store and like peas, you know, we shell peas coming out of the garden, out of the field garden, and tomatoes, we grow tomatoes. I remember, as tomatoes were growing I used to go out there practically every day just to see how tomatoes grow and how leaves develop and it was a beautiful sight to see, you know, 'cause each day it look like they would just develop and I always want to share that stuff when I always say, "When I have kids, I want to share that with my kids, you know . . . you don't have to have a whole bunch of money to survive."

For a small set of fathers, like Wyatt—who also talks about his family raising chickens and hogs—gardening is just one facet of a more traditional orientation toward living off the land by raising farm animals, hunting, and fishing.

Because I was every bit a grocery store kid with no gardening, hunting, or fishing experience, my mom's stories of what life was like living on a working farm in Pennsylvania with eight siblings is the primary means by which I came to know the rugged life of the farm family. I can still walk in my mind's eye through my grandma's cornfields, stare at fat pigs in messy stalls, pump and drink well water from a tin cup, play in a barn stacked full of hay bales, and use a dilapidated outhouse. Yet, like most adults and kids today, I am far removed from knowing experientially what this sort of life is truly like. My experience as a part-time dairy farm worker for six months in college gives me a glimmer of the life but not the deep feeling of the daily grind or personal connection to the land.

Food Shopping and Kitchen Culture

Food shopping is just one of many domestic chores that go along with running a household. In some instances, fathers excuse themselves or are excused by their partner from playing a major role in this activity. Some may be out of the shopping loop because they have demanding, time-consuming jobs that make it impractical for them to devote time to grocery shopping. Others may have a limited role because they have little to do with preparing family meals. But some dads say they do most of the food shopping and most say they do at least some of the shopping. The stay-at-home-dads certainly do the bulk of the shopping. For the dads who go grocery shopping, having kids with them is a fairly common routine, especially if the kids haven't started high school. However, just because the children are with their dads at the store doesn't mean that dads will use the outing as an opportunity to talk about nutrition. Unfortunately, only a small proportion of men see grocery shopping as a chance to create food shopping routines and rituals that accentuate health and fitness.

I can appreciate how some men may want to avoid the tense moments of warding off their kids' barrage of requests to buy certain foods. The tenor of my own shopping rituals with Phoenix changed once he became more demanding around the age of five or six. Depending on his mood, I struggle sometimes to keep our ritual upbeat and enjoyable while also directing him to healthy choices.

Brent not only promoted the garden experience for his kids but also took them grocery shopping when they were younger and had them think about dietary and nutritional issues as part of homeschooling lessons. They had to calculate the price and think about the nutritional value of different foods. He asked them to read labels and determine what was in different products.

Lewis, a certified personal trainer, is another father who capitalized on the grocery store experience and poured a lot of time and energy into teaching his son about the different facets of identifying and purchasing foods. He provides a detailed account of what he tried to accomplish with his now twenty-year-old son when they were both younger.

> Basically what I spoke about [was] staying out of cans, you don't wanna do too many canned items because, first of all, you don't know how long it's been sitting there just because there's a date on it. You wanna go with fresh. That conversation has primarily been about reading the labels, and if you do purchase something, read the labels on it. What's in it? If you're gonna get any boxed, or cereals, or anything like that, don't look at the front, let's look at the label, let's see what's inside, okay. And . . . instead of buying something where there's buying proprietary blends, where it just mentions a bunch of things and it doesn't give you an itemization, you probably don't wanna look at that one. So, I had him look at things that were gonna be itemized, where he could see specifically what nutritional items were in there from vitamins to minerals and so forth so he's getting the most for his money when he buys nutritional items. So a lot of it was based on reading labels, and what you're getting for your money, and trying to stay away from a lot of refined sugar type of stuff.

The tone of a food shopping trip varies widely among families, and individual trips can differ significantly depending on time and money constraints as well as what the shopping needs are on a given occasion—big weekly shop or a quick trip for a few items. Taking a young child, teenager, a child with special needs, or multiple children can alter the shopping dynamics as well.

An important characteristic of food shopping is the extent to which a father tends to be proactive and engaged in how he relates to his child. Does he see food shopping as a chance to pass on his values as a father or is it merely a domestic chore that needs to be accomplished as quickly and efficiently as possible? A father who has a heightened awareness about health and fitness is more likely to see shopping as an opportunity to be generative and pass on his values about the significance of what eating well means and how it can be achieved.

Fathers vary widely in their ability to absorb financially the costs of certain food choices whether they do the shopping or not. Whereas some are free to buy as much pricey organic food as they want, others must make strategic choices that are not always consistent with what they would like for their kids or themselves. Sometimes just figuring out a way to buy enough food to keep everyone's belly full proves to be a challenge.

Concerns about food costs come across clearly when listening to Jackson, a modestly paid thirty-year-old store clerk, describe the food shopping dilemma he encounters with his nine-year-old daughter and seven-year-old son, who split time between his place and their mother's home. Compared to his current cohabiting partner, this multiracial vegan dad has more patience and is willing to take the kids food shopping even though they are demanding and not as well-mannered as he would like at the store. When he shops with the kids, he tries to discuss nutrition with them, but he likes to move quickly through the store. With laughter in his voice he reenacts what his shopping conversations are usually like with his kids: "I always feel poor, so we'll go to the fruit section maybe and I'll say 'All right, what would you like?' and she always picks something that's not grown from here and costs a lot more and I'll say 'Sorry, why don't we stick to the apples? You can pick from these.'" By regularly taking the kids food shopping, Jackson is often reminded that his limited funds restrict his ability to fulfill his fathering aspirations.

Jackson firmly believes he could do better for his kids in food shopping if he made more money. For example, he would like to take them to the farmers' market more often and spend more money on food. Ideally, he would "like [to] get paid, go to the farmers' market, and just let them pick things that are healthy and then just to know that we have food just waiting for us and we never have to worry about it."

Unfortunately, unlike many fathers, who are free from the burden of having to coordinate shopping jaunts with their pay days, Jackson lives life week to week, paycheck to paycheck. He puts in perspective what life is like for many poor fathers: "When they're [his kids] here, we usually need food right then, so I get paid and we go to the store. Farmers' market isn't open when I get out of work." And even if the farmers' market were open,

Jackson feels constrained in how far he can stretch his meager wages to buy the food he would ideally like to have his children eat.

Although Jackson didn't explicitly describe himself as a locavore—a person who tries to eat only locally produced food—he seems to lean in that direction.[3] For example, every Wednesday he and his family receive a box of fruits and vegetables he orders online from a local farm, and he's also working on expanding his small family garden. Those who live most fully by the locavore philosophy are probably more likely to teach their children to be environmentally friendly in other ways as well. So dads of this ilk would tend to connect healthy eating with environmental consciousness for themselves and their children. In their eyes, passing these values on to children would be consistent with good fathering.

Despite the gradual cultural shift in the Western world concerning how good fathering is defined, breadwinning continues to be a critical dimension of how adult men, and others, perceive fathers' manliness and their value to their families—their children in particular.[4] The historical roots of the term "breadwinning" even emphasize a person's primary responsibility and ability to provide a staple of life—food—to one's family. Not being able to buy the kinds of food one thinks one's children should have can carry the same stigma and pain as not being able to provide them with the medicines or medical procedures they need to thrive physically.

Grover, an African American father in his early fifties, is reminded constantly of his limited resources when he spends time in a grocery store. His life is littered with a series of struggles that have contributed to his financial problems: he is a high school dropout who failed ninth grade four times, a drug addict, in and out of prison many times, and is now disabled and unemployed. He illustrates how his lack of money guides his thinking while shopping for food.

> I buy a pack of pork chops right, what I do, I count up every pork chop in the pack and then I count up everybody in the house so everybody gets a piece of meat, you know, and I try to get the cheapest thing that I can where everybody can have some. And the cheapest thing you can get is really not the best thing good for you, for your health. You know, chicken the same way. We eat a lot of chicken. We eat a lot of pork chops, because that's really the cheapest thing that's on the market.

Fathers, whether they are strapped for money, middle-income, or wealthy, can try to educate their kids about proper nutrition. For the dads who strive to educate their kids about nutrition at the grocery store or elsewhere it's always nice to know that the kids are actually listening and affected. The physician Jonathan, with twenty- and seventeen-year-old sons, describes how he and his wife frequently took the boys to the grocery store when they were younger and would "explain the differences between the different foods and the different fats, the good fats, bad fats monounsaturated, polyunsaturated, you know looking at the different calories, protein versus carbohydrate, we'd make a pretty good educational trip when we went." He continues by mentioning that his kids now use Fooducate, a phone app that allows a user to photograph the barcode in order to generate a grade, which is displayed, representing the quality of the product in terms of the amount of carbohydrates, proteins, fat, and the like. He feels "pretty good" knowing that his kids use the app. Although he chuckles when speculating that they will "default to Taco Bell if they have a choice," he acknowledges that "they've gotten to be smarter shoppers and smarter about food."

Grocery stores and farmers' markets are important sites that afford parents opportunities to engage their children in talks about nutrition, but fathers can talk to their kids about nutrition just about anywhere. Preparing food in the kitchen and eating family meals together are two additional and obvious settings where such talks can naturally emerge.

Plenty of parenting experts provide advice for parents struggling to get their children to eat their fruits and vegetables, and scholarly research documents the difficulties many parents have.[5] Not surprisingly, research shows that compared to families who never have meals together, families who eat many or all of their meals together are much more likely to have children who frequently consume fruits and vegetables. Although researchers can't say for sure what it is about eating meals together that matters, it seems plausible that parental supervision comes into play.

Cadel, a thirty-five-year-old of Jamaican and Chinese descent, is big on having family meal time with his wife and their four children, all under ten years of age. As the primary cook in the family he shares his secret for getting his kids to eat their vegetables: "I'll cook up a spread that they'll love, but I said, 'Here everybody, come to the kitchen, handful of carrots. If you want the rest of your food, eat your handful of carrots.'"

Reflecting on their childhood experiences, fathers offer widely varying accounts of what the kitchen culture was like in their family and
how involved they were in it. Their experiences ranged from completely
detached and uninterested to intense involvement in all aspects of meal
preparation. Some played a prominent role in acquiring food through gardening, hunting, fishing, or grocery store shopping. While at least three-
quarters witnessed their fathers doing some of the cooking or grilling, only
a small minority witnessed their fathers taking a primary role in preparing
meals for them. Consistent with national trends, the generations of fathers
I interviewed generally do more cooking than their fathers did for them.[6]

At one end of the spectrum for food preparation is Ricardo, a
fifty-one-year-old Cuban adoptive father. He describes himself as not helping in the kitchen at all during his youth, in part because he was well aware
that his father expected him not to be involved in kitchen matters. His father
perceived kitchen activities as a feminine domain. Ricardo did not challenge those views until he was away at college. Other men's limited involvement in meal preparation was rooted in their fundamental lack of interest,
often connected to their longing for a lifestyle they felt provided them far
more exciting leisure opportunities.

As I reflect on my own childhood experience I'm well aware now, as I
superficially was during my youth, that Dad did not do any cooking or bak-
ing. On rare occasions, he made a few sandwiches with me, but I don't ever
recall him using the stove or microwave while I lived at home. I'm sure his
lack of involvement influenced my lack of interest in knowing what was happening on the cooking front, and I suspect that the prevailing norms of the
1960s and 1970s about what "real" boys and men should be doing factored
into my rudimentary thinking as well.

A fair number of dads recall helping out as kids by doing minor food
preparation tasks because they were asked to do so, or in some cases
because they wanted to get involved. Turning to their own practices with
their children, some fathers actively try to promote their children's involvement in the kitchen.

When Lewis's son Prince was ten or eleven he began to take an interest
in what Lewis was doing in the kitchen. But there was a period of time that
Prince didn't want to have much or anything to do with the kitchen. Lewis
worked to motivate Prince by making him special meals and then asking

him how much he liked them. When Prince said he really liked something, Lewis would ask if he wanted to learn how to make it. The strategy worked.

Cadel is committed to preparing family dinners as well as desserts for his wife and kids. He describes himself as the "big homemade guy" and makes sure that his kids know this about him. Whenever possible he gets the kids involved in preparing meals because doing so jibes with his philosophy about instilling a sense of responsibility to their family and for their own choices. When he makes pancakes, "they're full on, like they'll come in, put everything in to mix the pancakes, then one person gets to stir, one person gets to add this teaspoon, one person gets to add this cup. At the end of it, they get to, maybe, drop one ladle full of pancake batter on the griddle." Making pancakes into a family affair has apparently swayed the kids to appreciate the joy of cooking: they love and frequently watch the Food Network channel on their own.

By integrating his kids into his family's kitchen culture, Cadel limits the sacrifices he might otherwise have to make in order to devote time to his kids. However, for some dads, especially those with infants or whose children have time-consuming extracurricular agendas, asserting themselves in the kitchen may require critical choices about how much time they spend doing things with and for their kids. When kids are not intimately involved in making dinners, a father's time spent making homemade lasagna, for instance, can pull him away from other activities with his children. Thus, nurturing dads must consider the pros and cons of preparing homemade meals and spending less time with their children versus resorting to frozen dinners or eating out and spending more time with them. Some dads can deal with these time management issues if they jointly prepare meals with their partners or take turns making meals throughout the week. If circumstances permit, combining kitchen time with kid time is clearly the ideal.

PHILOSOPHIES OF COOKING, FOOD, DIET, AND BODY IMAGE

We can appreciate fathers' and children's experiences with food and health more clearly by placing them in a larger cultural context. The food culture of a home is often influenced by a family's commitment to upholding religious and ethnic philosophies that dictate the meaning of cooking and eating as well as practical food choices. Scholars who study different social groups and their approach to food focus on "foodways": "eating habits and culinary practices of a people, region, or historical period."[7] Identifying distinct foodways and making sense of how they matter for individuals is challenging in a multicultural, dynamic, and regionally diverse society like the United States.[8] In addition, the everyday realities associated with migration and economic disadvantage can alter how ethnic communities and families adapt to their less than ideal circumstances. With due caution, I briefly illustrate the potential significance of a few notable foodways and social forces that can affect fathers and their children.

My Latin acquaintances repeatedly share stories about being immersed in an ethnic community that reinforces expectations for eating a lot. Those stories are echoed in the experiences of Rafael, one of the men I interviewed. Now forty-eight, he vividly recalls a "very unhappy" period during his adolescence when he gained a lot of weight at age thirteen. Rafael felt "very troubled" by his condition because his friends were in better shape than he was. After doing research at a library to learn about his body and dieting, he changed his diet on his own by cutting out the "starches and the carbs and the fats." During the first several months he trimmed down considerably and felt much better. He sustained his focused dieting for a year and a half. In a disappointed tone, however, he recalls how his family failed to respond as well as his friends did to his weight loss. When I ask him why, he reasons, "You have to understand that [in] Cuban cultures, chubby is the norm." Although Rafael freely admits that Cuban cuisine is "really good tasting," he's also aware of the health issues linked to the style of cooking he's experienced. Thus, he closely monitors his consumption of Cuban food.

While Latinos may be inclined to eat food in large quantities, diet and health professionals actually view traditional Latin American foodways as ideal because they emphasize maize, beans, rice, and fresh fruit and vegetables as well as a the preparation of fresh meals and many kinds of food.[9] Because Latinos may be more inclined to sit down in the company of friends and family for meals, they are also less likely to eat alone or eat on the go—patterns associated with unwanted weight gain. Unfortunately, these traditional foodways are in decline for many people of Latin descent living in America.

The increased health problems of Latinos in the United States related to obesity, diabetes, and hypertension appear to be linked to the food habits they have adopted since migrating to America. Zilkia Janer, a professor of global studies and geography, argues that migration patterns that have relocated Latinos to urban areas leave them with limited access to land, which prevents them from growing fresh fruits and vegetables even though many have the skills to do so. Consequently, they are more likely to rely on processed foods and have substituted fast foods for more traditional choices. The eating habits of men and fathers who are migratory workers isolated in labor camps are adversely affected because they often have limited cooking facilities and don't have the means to travel to grocery stores. Additionally, middle-class Latinos have their own difficulties as more and more adopt mainstream American eating habits and begin to consume their richer traditional dishes more regularly.[10]

Although Latin women have traditionally assumed cooking responsibilities in the United States and Latin America, an increasing number of Latin men are acquiring cooking skills by working in restaurant kitchens where they experiment with all sorts of cuisines. If these skills allow Latin fathers to contribute more directly to their families' daily food culture, their increased presence in the kitchen is likely to alter their children's perceptions about food preparation as well as their eating habits.

Culinary arts and food science professor Jonathan Deutsch provides another example of the possible influence of an ethnic foodway on fathers and children. He notes that "many traditional Jewish foods, especially from the Ashkenazi diet, are full of nutritional red flags: few fresh fruits and vegetables, low in fiber, high in fat, high in refined flours and sugars."[11] Viewed from a historical lens, the traditional Ashkenazic cuisine is not so much a by-product of modern American Jewish culture per se; rather, it stems from the poor living conditions and food options that defined the lives of the generations of Jews who migrated to the United States from eastern Europe. The end result, though, is that Ashkenazi Jews tend to have elevated rates of irritable bowel syndrome, Crohn's disease, and ulcerative colitis that appear to be related in part to their diet. Such patterns can place children in a precarious position when they are swept up in the everyday food rituals of their fathers and other elders. Fortunately, young Jewish children may be at less risk for negative health outcomes than earlier generations because the

traditional Jewish American diet is in decline as "health-conscious preparations and styles of cooking" become more appealing. In addition, different
food companies as well as community groups are beginning to support new
and healthier recipes for traditional Jewish foods.[12]

Although the growing diversity of Jewish American families has led to
a dramatic reduction in the number of traditional domestic arrangements,
many families still identify the woman as the principal person in charge of
food preparation, irrespective of employment status. In these households,
the Jewish father, like his children, may be a somewhat passive bystander in
his ethnic food culture. However, in recent years, as more Jewish women—
even those who are traditional and observant—enter the workplace, they
are beginning to share cooking duties, including preparations for the Shab-
bat and holiday meals.[13] As this occurs, Jewish fathers may begin to play a
more prominent role in making dietary decisions that affect themselves as
well as their children.

Whatever foodway and ethnic cuisine is being scrutinized, there's no
straightforward relationship between specific foodways and obesity. Trying
to disentangle how much a particular ethnic diet matters above and beyond
the influence of other related conditions, such as, exercise and leisure
patterns, income, and genetics is tricky. The story is also complicated when
viewed from an international perspective because commentators often
point to how the American fast food tradition of eating has raised obesity
rates in various countries that have historically had healthier food habits.[14]

In addition to the foodways typically associated with particular ethnic
groups, vegan and vegetarian philosophies are other types of traditions that
shape people's perceptions of food, nutrition, and cooking habits. Those
who adopt these perspectives may also be influenced by aspects of other
ethnic and regional foodways. Like individuals affected by the typical foodways, many vegans and vegetarians personally see themselves as being associated with a group identity. Each of the dads I spoke with who practiced
one of these alternative foodways was quite conscious about his own and
his children's experiences with food and eating. By being different from the
mainstream, these fathers often face a unique set of issues with managing
their children's eating practices at home and in public.

Despite the potential challenges that alternative foodways can present,
when a father with minor children adopts such a philosophy, he may positively influence his child's short- and long-term health, because meatless

diets are associated with a lower body mass index, lower blood pressure, and a reduced risk of type 2 diabetes.[15] A father with this profile may also be more likely to consider himself to be a locavore. He may involve his children in family rituals that include visits to farmers' markets or community-supported agriculture (CSA) projects.[16]

PHYSICAL ACTIVITY

One of the more amazing and inspiring stories a dad shared with me about a family ritual was Brent's description of how he and his father cycled on their ten-speeds two hours a day, at least five days a week, for roughly six straight years, beginning when Brent was in the fourth or fifth grade. They would get up at four o'clock and be on their bikes by four-thirty. Their exploratory rides often took them into new residential developments and roads. As he recalls, "Some mornin's we would talk, we would ride real slow and we'd just jibber jabber the whole way and some mornin's we would just ride as hard and fast as we could and we wouldn't say a word." He laughs as he notes how the ritual came to an end when his high school sports, long days, and homework led him to reason, "No more was I getting up at four o'clock in the mornin.'"

That Brent faithfully got out of bed for years at four in the morning during his youth in order to exercise with his dad is remarkable. That he stopped the ritual in high school is understandable. His commitment as a kid speaks volumes about his love for his dad and the reciprocal nature of many successful family rituals. A child's level of cooperation and enthusiasm will go a long way in determining whether a mundane routine becomes a meaningful ritual. A father may be willing to invest his time, energy, and sweat in exercising with his child, but if he has to beg, cajole, or threaten the child to make it happen he might decide that it isn't worth the hassle. The same applies to any health- or fitness-related venture a father might try to establish.

I often wonder how far I should push Phoenix to do joint physical activities with me. Left to his own devices and unmonitored, Phoenix will more often than not choose to play inside with toys or video games. But once he's in motion he thrives at playing numerous sports outside in the yard or on competitive teams. He also loves swimming and mountain biking through the woods and neighborhoods, generally enjoys training on his road bike, and tolerates running. He even on occasion gets into landscaping projects that require his muscles or digging abilities. The trick, then, is to get him into the flow and immersed in an outdoor activity.

In the presence of other kids, Phoenix is likely to go full throttle, but he is sometimes less motivated without the playmate incentive. This may be typical for kids his age. However, I often imagine how I would have responded to growing up on the property I own now. If other kids were not around, how much time would I have spent outdoors playing either by myself or only with my dad? Growing up, I longed to play in an open field and explore the woods. I also never walked away from the sporting activities I did with my dad; he was always the one to call it quits.

I have tried to make Phoenix's home environment sports-friendly, with an adjustable hoop and glass backboard in the driveway, a soccer field, and different bikes and sports equipment in the garage. When Phoenix was seven, I arranged a family membership at a pool so that he and I could swim laps. I've also worked at creating different rituals—"sports dates"—to bring his friends to the house to practice basketball, football, soccer, and baseball or to run around playing dodgeball and kickball. Playing pool games and arranging biking excursions with other kids and dads has been part of the recreational menu as well. Signing him up for different sports activities provides some structure to his life and has helped to get him outdoors or into a gym. Finally, for the after-school pickup, I've resorted to getting water bottles ready in advance, having a change of clothes in the car, and our bikes loaded on the car to circumvent any need to go inside the house or tendency to succumb to sedentary temptations. Am I overzealous about the dark side of laziness—too eager to teach healthy habits for the body and instill an appreciation for outside activities? Perhaps—but I would rather err on the side of exercise and time spent in nature.

I was amused to hear that Jonathan resorted to treating joint exercise with his kids as a unique form of discipline. He describes having a number of "attitude runs"—mostly with his younger son. This was his way of connecting with his boys and trying to get them to come to see precisely what they had done wrong when they misbehaved. He jokingly says though that as his youngest son got bigger and faster the runs turned out to be more of a punishment for him, the father.

As Jonathan's example suggests, not all rituals are deemed enjoyable by both the father and the child who participates in them. So too, some rituals with potential health and fitness benefits may actually be designed to achieve a different kind of outcome. Some rituals are clearly influenced by how a dad's style of fathering guides his approach to a health-related activity.

Those who do research in the exercise sciences and related fields tend to look at five broad types of circumstances that influence kids' level of physical activity: biological (age, sex), cognitive (goal orientation, intention), behavioral (sports involvement), social (parent modeling, others' support), and physical environment (availability of parks, gyms, fields).[17] Some research looks at how fathers and mothers contribute to children's physical activity (PA) levels. Parents can provide encouragement, be involved and model active physical behavior, and facilitate activities (transportation, registration fees) that enable children to participate in organized sports. A key assumption often implied in this research is that more active parents will have more active children who are less likely to be obese.

Although findings are mixed, most studies find that higher parental activity levels are correlated with kids' higher physical activity levels, although parental support may actually be the critical force shaping kids' activity levels. Several research teams have concluded that fathers tend to make a difference in their children's weight outcomes separate from whatever influence mothers may have.[18]

Being proactive is an important aspect of a father supporting his child's physical activity. Identifying possible recreational sports in the community, buying equipment, and suggesting that a kid experiment with a particular sport and practice it are ways fathers can make a difference in children's openness to exercise.

In recent decades, a dad's involvement in his child's sports participation has taken on new meaning because it's connected to a wider set of complex changes in youth sports, family ideology, and family life. Jay Coakley, a sociologist who studies the social dimensions of sports, argues that youth sports have been transformed by becoming "increasingly privatized, regionally located, expensive, performance-oriented, and highly structured in terms of participation schedules."[19] As a result, contemporary kids are much more dependent on their parents to help them get and stay involved. Coakley also points to how the changing cultural expectation that parents be more accountable for their children's actions and whereabouts has led to parents feeling more responsible for when their kids fail or succeed in sports. In particular, youth sports increasingly provide dads, especially those among the middle and upper-middle classes, fresh opportunities to be involved in their children's lives in nurturing, more publicly visible ways.

Fathers in recent decades have also been exposed to a cultural climate that increasingly supports girls' participation in organized sports even though the "pattern of gender relations across family, school, and community still favors athletic options for boys more so than girls."[20] One consequence of this gendered pattern is revealed in a 2007 national study that surveyed students in grades 3 through 12 as well as parents of other children in these grades. It shows that boys are much more likely than girls to list their dads as teaching them the most about exercise and sports play, 46 percent to 28 percent, respectively.[21] Reports from the parental survey reinforce this finding, with fewer fathers than mothers saying that they would know "what steps to take" to "help a girl get more physically active." As we move deeper into the next few decades this gender gap may narrow if women increasingly enter motherhood with an athletic background, but the data suggest that boys continue to have more opportunities than girls to compete in organized sports.[22] Anecdotally, my own six years of coaching several youth sports in north central Florida also leaves me with the impression that the dads are more active than the moms in teaching my players about the sports I coach. And although I didn't systematically compare how much the dads I spoke with were involved in promoting their daughters' versus sons' physical activity, I got the impression that many dads promoted some form of physical activity for their daughters.

Like me, many men choose to get engaged in their children's sports activities by volunteering to coach. When dads coach their relatively young (elementary school) children they often choose between or end up juggling two contrasting models of masculinity that shape their style of fathering.[23] One is based on a more orthodox form of masculinity and is tied to a performance ethos, whereas the other is connected to a more inclusive, progressive form of masculinity and a nurturing style of fathering. In our contemporary culture, more dads are trying to incorporate aspects of the inclusive approach even if they also expect their kids to learn skills, perform well, and try to win. Regardless of the model of masculinity they express, dads increasingly are valuing the intimate space and moments they can share with their children in various sports settings, sometimes prioritizing this form of play over their work responsibilities. However, the new norms that encourage dads to be more nurturing toward their children both in and away from a sports environment are compelling men to doubt themselves as fathers as they try to balance their competitive, pressure-laden investments in youth sports with their caring, supportive efforts. Today, dads who take an active role in their children's sports, whether as coaches or highly supportive fans, may be more introspective about their style of fathering. Will their intense approach inadvertently push kids to drop out of sports as they move into middle school and beyond? I sometimes personally wrestle with this question while I manage the serious training Phoenix does as a competitive triathlete.

In their book *Young Athletes, Couch Potatoes, and Helicopter Parents: The Productivity of Play*, Jessica Skolnikoff and Robert Engvall discuss how dad-coaches in youth sports affect their child's chances to succeed in this arena.[24] They extend Malcolm Gladwell's conclusions in his 2008 best seller *Outliers* that those who are truly standouts in a field develop their talent through the connections they often make at a young age, the increased practice time they get, and the specialized coaching they receive. Skolniknoff and Engvall agree with Gladwell's basic idea, but they encourage us to understand that many kids who are labeled "standouts" benefit from an initial and subtle selection process that implicates them as the "chosen ones." These kids are given unique opportunities and tend to be given greater latitude to fail as they gain experience. Not surprisingly, kids who excel at sports are more likely to continue in their athletic endeavors and in many instances incur the benefits associated with regular, vigorous exercise.

This observation resonates with me because Phoenix and I share plenty of time doing drills and planning basketball practice sessions prior to a season and a game. Consequently, I talk to Phoenix extensively on and off the court about my coaching philosophy, the value of drills, specific plays, and strategies for building team chemistry. I afford him numerous opportunities to run the team as a point guard, partly because he has learned what all the players on the court are supposed to do on specific plays. In addition, as a coach's son he has learned that he has unique opportunities to help his teammates in various ways and demonstrate leadership qualities. As a result, on a good day, he feels invested in the team and committed to exercise. I trust that the opportunities I'm giving Phoenix will encourage him to adopt a long-term, healthy approach to sport and fitness more generally as well as more confidence in his leadership abilities.

AN EYE ON SAFETY

It was a pleasant autumn Saturday afternoon in Mansfield, Pennsylvania. Now a junior in college, I had emerged from my basement "study cave" in my apartment to hang out with Scott. "Scooter," "Scooter, where are you?" I playfully called as I checked for my two-and-a half-year-old son in my apartment's several rooms. By the time I reached the living room, the last of the potential hiding places, my playful mood turned to confusion. My son and I were *not* supposed to be playing a game of hide-and-seek. Where was he?

I asked his mother, who was standing in the kitchen, where he was. Her "I don't know" reply and puzzled look shifted me to concern. A quick look on the front porch came up empty, but the screen door that I wanted locked at all times was not. "Scott, Scott, Scott!" I yelled from the front porch. I bolted down three wooden stairs, turned right, and jogged down the side-walk toward the small pizza shop next door. No sign of him in the empty parking lot, so I picked up my pace with my head on a swivel. "Scott, Scott, where are you?" my voice now in a full scream, my heart pounding, a ner-vous energy overtook me. To the back street I hurried, turning right to go alongside the house that was behind my apartment. I frantically made my way up the sidewalk to the small backyard where Scott and I had played in his toddler pool a few months earlier. I checked in the detached wooden garage and looked in my green Mercury Capri, which sat in the driveway. I heard his mother's voice calling for him on the other side of the house. No sign of my son—I was in panic mode. "What's going on, where's my little boy?" I thought to myself. Tears welled in my eyes.

I ran to the front of the house to redo my search. This time, I went across the narrow street into the neighbors' front yard calling, "Scott! Scott, where are you?" A head of wavy blond hair popped out of a sizable mound of large red maple leaves. "Scott, what are you doing? You can't leave the house!" I exclaimed as I swooped him up into my arms. I cuddled him to my chest. My hand cupped his head, pressing it tightly into the nape of my neck. "You scared Daddy. I didn't know where you were!" I wasn't letting go anytime soon.

As I stood there, rocking Scooter in my arms, my fear faded from my conscious mind. But, unbeknownst to me, the sensory overload that marked my fright during those seemingly endless few minutes had etched itself deep into my subconscious. The results of that primal process is akin to how the scent of musky, dampness instantly triggers my childhood memories to reconstruct images of the time I spent in the upstairs bedrooms in my grandmother's early twentieth-century farmhouse.

With the passing of time, and Scott's increasing maturity, I became oblivious to the memories I forged on that autumn afternoon. Phoenix's birth, and his increasing mobility during infancy, changed all of that. I rediscovered the neural network that encoded my fear of losing a child, feelings that were augmented by my concerns about my child's safety more generally. Scott's mischievous legacy included another decisive moment: I had disturbing long-term memories of speeding up to ninety miles an hour on a narrow, rural highway after receiving news at my part-time job on a dairy farm that my toddler son Scott might have poisoned himself by eating Vaseline. Despite being reassured by his mother upon my arrival home that all should be fine, the numbing memories persist of what might have been.

So, when Phoenix was born I was quick to baby-proof the house, especially the doorknobs. In public spaces I vigilantly kept Phoenix within reach whether other family members were around or not, and without exception I carried him or held his hand in parking lots and crowded places. Although a few relatives found my protective style of keeping close tabs on Phoenix over the top and off-putting, I was determined to do what I believed any good father should do—keep his vulnerable child's best interests in clear view by following one simple rule: plan for the worst and hope for the best.

On Christmas Eve 2012, I deliberately stepped back from my protective fathering. Phoenix, my wife, and I were doing our annual walk at an elaborate holiday light display at a small pond connected to the hospital complex where Phoenix was born. My wife was in the center holding hands with Phoenix and me. A snowman balloon exhibit caught Phoenix's attention and he pulled away to check it out. He then casually walked in front of us on the circular path as he took in the festive scenery and music. As usual, the place was crowded with families and romantic couples. I was tempted

to call Phoenix back to my side, but I resisted. My "self-talk" kicked in—
"Relax, it can be okay. Just enjoy Kendra's company for the moment—this
is an intimate and romantic setting. He's right there. He's okay. It's okay."

"I don't see him. Do you see him? Where is he?" I exclaimed to Kendra.
In what seemed like a blink of any eye, Phoenix had disappeared. When I
lunged forward to search my inner voice berated me, "You idiot! Why didn't
you grab his hand! You never let him wander about in public. Why now?"
"Phoenix, Phoenix, Phoenix!" I called his name into the sea of dimly lit
faces and colorful Christmas decorations. No answer. I circled each exhibit I
came to and moved ahead as quickly as I could. Images of Scott going missing flooded my brain. I knew this intense, consuming fear all too well. And
this time it seemed worse: I was outside my neighborhood and it was dark.

New tears welled in my eyes while I circled the pond with no sign of
Phoenix, or my wife for that matter. In my panic, I had rushed out in front
of her, needing to go at my own pace.

Minutes later and halfway around the pond on my second lap, I ran into
my family. I embraced Phoenix much as I had done with Scott decades
earlier. I sat him down in the grass, gave him a firm lecture on safety issues
in public places, and told him his poor choice had scared me to "infinity
and beyond."

Many parents can relate to my stories. They can recite their own rendition that captures the shock, fear, and perhaps sadness they absorbed during some noteworthy difficult moment of raising their kids. Sometimes
those stories gain national notoriety, such as when the nineteen-year-old
son of retired legendary professional basketball player Julius Erving (Dr. J.)
went missing in 2000. His car and body were found five long weeks later in
a pond near the family home. The death was ruled an accidental drowning.
Fortunately, many tales have happier endings that subsequently get woven
into a family's folklore, "Do you remember that time when . . . ?"

But far too many parents like Dr. J. are left with tears that flow for days,
weeks, months, and sometimes years after they learn that their child has
been seriously harmed or injured in some way, received a dire medical diagnosis, or gone missing for an extended period of time. Some are plagued by
regrets that they could have, should have done more to prevent the tragedy
that damaged their child's life, or perhaps even took it.

Because I spoke with a diverse set of fathers I heard unfortunate stories
about all sorts of "bad news" health events. They mainly included physical

accidents and unfavorable medical tests, but I also heard about molestation, abortion, and drug overdosing. Many of these events forever changed their children's quality of life. I delve deeply into fathers' experiences with chronic illnesses and conditions in later chapters but I begin here to reveal fathers' efforts to protect their children and to keep them out of harm's way.

Bad news events are often tied to the world of risk taking. Kids are exposed to various types of risks during their formative years. Some risks, such as an accidental gun shooting in the home, can be easily controlled or eliminated; others, like falling off a bike, less so. Some risks—for example, chemical poisoning—have immediate, perceptible consequences, while others can produce negative consequences that only appear years later—think of skin cancer from excessive sun exposure. Doing a belly flop off a diving board carries relatively minor consequences; driving without a seatbelt can have life-altering or fatal results. Some risks—recklessly driving a motorcycle a hundred miles per hour, especially without a helmet—are reasonably well understood by youth and adults alike; others may be largely misunderstood by youth and even some parents—using prescription painkillers comes to mind. In many respects, what is most important is how fathers perceive risks rather than the objective odds of something happening.

The more devastating examples of child tragedies—many of which can be interpreted through a risk-taking lens—are regularly depicted and recycled in the entertainment and news media. The news media's 24/7 coverage of horrific stories that connect kids to guns, car accidents, poisonings, kidnappings, physical abuse, and the like has escalated parental worrying in recent decades. Paradoxically, while many parents often have exaggerated perceptions of the odds that certain bad things will happen to their child, many parents and their children mistakenly think that specific bad outcomes will only happen to someone else.[25]

With the help of some basic facts, let's put into perspective several well-known childhood tragedies that can influence fathers' perceptions and choices. Annually, three million kids, a number that exceeds the entire population of Chicago, are treated in emergency rooms in the United States because of accidental injuries that happen at home. Each year, roughly 2,100 children age fourteen and younger die from accidental injuries in the home.[26] Most of these deaths are the result of fire, suffocation, drowning, choking, a fall, poisoning, or firearms.

Between 2008 and 2010, the numbers of children from birth to age nineteen who died because of an unintentional firearm injury, homicide, and suicide, were 371, 5,665, and 5,693, respectively. From 2010 through 2012, more than 15,000 children were treated for gun-related injuries.[27]

Numbers, of course, only tell part of the story. In the spring of 2013, the national spotlight was directed at Caroline Sparks, a two-year-old girl from southern Kentucky, and her family.[28] One afternoon, when the mother briefly stepped outside their home, Caroline's five-year-old brother accidentally shot her in the chest and killed her with the .22 caliber Crickett rifle he was given for his birthday. The single-shot rifle, which comes in various bright colors and swirls, is directly marketed to kids.

This incident, like many others involving children, spurred the usual gun control debates on the Internet, television, and radio focusing on a range of issues including parental judgment and supervision, or the lack thereof. As of 2013, a Gallup Poll found that 42 percent of American adults have a gun on their property.[29] Because men are twice as likely as women to report personally owning a gun (46 to 23 percent), the culture of gun ownership and use is much more about what men—many of whom are fathers—think and do.[30] Clearly, millions of children live with their fathers or visit them in homes where a gun is stored. Thus millions of children are potentially vulnerable to unfortunate circumstances when fathers act irresponsibly while managing guns.

Cars, not guns, are the biggest cause of death for teenagers. About 2,163 teens ages sixteen to nineteen were killed in 2013 in motor vehicle accidents. Another 243,243 were treated and released from emergency care because of injuries suffered in motor-vehicle crashes. Teens have the lowest rate of always using seatbelts when they ride with someone else, 55 percent, compared to other age groups. Teens also are more likely than older drivers to speed, and their risk of being in a motor vehicle crash is greater at all levels of blood alcohol concentration. Male teen drivers and their passengers are almost twice as likely as their female counterparts to be involved in a fatal car wreck.[31]

When speaking to me, the dads who comment on seat belt use are adamant that they require their kids to use their belts. The reality, though, is that kids are free to make their own choices when they are driving or riding without a parent in the car. Getting those safety messages to stick when dads and moms are not around is vital.

Based merely on calls to the National Capital Poison Center for 2013, 16,655 children under six years of age were exposed to a poison, and there are likely far more incidents of children coming into contact with poisons that are not reported to this center.[32] Several of the most common substances include cosmetics/personal care products, pain medications, and cleaners. Fewer but more serious poison exposures occurred in adolescents. Each of these incidents has a story and many implicate fathers in one way or another.

One of Dustin's bad news stories unfolded when he came home from work in the afternoon to find his three-year-old son, Tommy, slurring words. Fortunately, Tommy was able to tell Dustin, "I don't feel good. I took some of mommy's pills." Dustin later found out that Tommy had climbed on top of his mother's dresser and found the bottle of pills she takes for epilepsy. After Dustin rushed Tommy to the hospital the boy remained there for three weeks. "He was even so bad that they had to put some kind of cap over his head with wires sticking out of it. . . . Tommy was fried . . . He didn't wake up for like a week!" Dustin was "so pissed" at his wife that he confronted her harshly for not properly securing her medication. He even went so far as to say, "I swear to God, if you were a man right now, I'd take you out in the yard and I would beat your ass." Fortunately, this bad news story has an encouraging ending: Tommy shows no lasting effects of his overdose four years ago.

To look closely at "bad news" health scenarios with an eye on fathers and their kids, we must see the scenarios against a cultural backdrop in which people increasingly perceive the fast-paced, media-saturated world as a dangerous place to raise kids. Many of the older fathers nostalgically reflected on their boyhood days during the 1960s, 1970s, and 1980s when they roamed freely on foot, bikes, and subways. It was not uncommon for some raised during these times, like me, to take off from their homes and sometimes neighborhoods for much of the day only to return for food, and perhaps a little cash. Fears of the lurking "bad man"—what is now called stranger danger—were not as deeply ingrained into the public's thinking about parenting.

Without ever giving it a second thought, and with my fairly strict parents knowing what I was doing, I regularly hitchhiked as a teenager in the early 1970s to the community pool a few miles from my home. But years later, I didn't want Scott doing anything similar, nor will I condone Phoenix hitch-hiking when he ventures out on his own.

As John Walsh's heart-wrenching story reveals, the climate for raising kids has changed considerably since I was a boy. A hotel developer in 1981, Walsh's life began to unravel when his six-year-old son, Adam, was abducted from a mall near his home in Hollywood, Florida. Two weeks later, Adam's severed head was found in a canal 120 miles away from the mall. In subsequent years, Walsh has channeled his anguish by making it his life's mission to catch the bad guys. With that mission in mind, Walsh created and hosted two television shows, *America's Most Wanted* and, more recently, *The Hunt with John Walsh*. He is also the cofounder of the National Center for Missing and Exploited Children. These initiatives have helped to resolve numerous missing child cases, but some see Walsh's efforts as controversial because they have led to a distorted perception of the pervasiveness of child kidnappings by strangers.

Even though thirty-nine-year-old Emmit, a father of two boys ages eleven and sixteen, was one of the more cautious dads I interviewed, many fathers embrace some version of his sentiment about kids and public safety. In our exchange about what he does with his sons when they're out of school and he and his wife are at work, Emmit turns particularly pensive and expresses his concerns about letting his kids play outside. "'Cause I'm so a-afraid of like you know just so many, like sexual predators and you don't know who is watching your house these days and stuff, and we live in an apartment complex and you know, and that's one of the places where you usually see people that, just released from like an institution or something like that, or incarcerated, you know like, easily can move into versus living in a neighborhood and stuff." Unfortunately, the combination of Emmit's work schedule, his wife's work hours, his stranger-dangers fears, and his views about his own neighborhood's risk potential makes for a potent mix of circumstances that confine his boys to house activities for many hours a week. In the winter, when daylight is scarce, the boys' outside physical activities are limited even more.

Although the real probability of a bad man (or woman) abusing a child is exaggerated in the public's mind, sometimes a man with bad intentions does enter into a child's life. When this happens, fathers often find themselves called upon to step up and be supportive. This happened when a martial arts instructor molested Greer's elementary school daughter.

Greer, a thirty-eight-year-old former service member who was deployed twice to combat duty in Iraq and Afghanistan, was recently divorced at the time he discovered what had happened to his daughter months earlier. Greer struggled to navigate this sensitive situation with a coparent who had a boyfriend and was not willing to act on Greer's suggestion that they seek counseling for the girl. He was especially worried that the unseen consequences of this trauma would surface later in life and affect his daughter's mental and emotional health. But as a nonresident father he deferred to his ex-wife's judgment and hoped for the best because he did not want to press the issue and stress out his daughter.

As someone who prided himself on being a man who protected his family, he took the news particularly hard. "I was blown away. . . . Of course as a dad I wanted to see this man, ya know, hurt [laughs] bad, but, of course we let the legal system, go through its course." Greer delicately spoke to his daughter initially to figure out which of the instructors was responsible but he didn't talk to her much about the incident the first year after it occurred. Over the last several years he has discussed the situation with her a bit. "I sat down with her and I said, 'Okay, you realize that what happened was not appropriate. You realize that by me putting you in that environment, I feel like it was my fault. Like I put you in a situation, where you were left [in] after school care, you're pretty much in the hands of some strangers.'"

Greer has, to some extent, been able to relate to what his daughter experienced because he was molested as a kid by his mother's boyfriend. He was frustrated that the "evil" repeated itself in his family. In some ways his own molestation experience accentuates his guilt and aggravation over not being able to "fix" the situation for his daughter.

Just as Emmit exemplifies the intensely cautious kind of dad, Greer provides a glimpse of what a father is like who confides that he sees himself distinctly as a protector of the home. As an ex-combat marine and former deputy sheriff, he personally knows what it's like to force himself into another person's home. Troubled by PTSD and nightmares, he frequently draws upon his professional experience to think about how he would react if someone broke into his apartment, a place where he is supposed to be in control.

RISK CULTURE

We can also dissect the larger cultural context by focusing on the way risk taking is expressed as part of a parenting style that typically differs between fathers and mothers. As we learn from Andrea Doucet's interviews with 118 primary-caregiver dads, some of whom are stay-at-home-dads, fathers are more likely than mothers to interact with their children in ways that expose their children to calculated risk taking in settings inside and outside the home.[33] Fathers are also more likely to encourage their children's independence in achieving certain developmental tasks—some of which carry the initial risk of failure.

This pattern resonates with me: I consistently push Phoenix to stretch his comfort zone in fitness-related activities involving the pool, playground, athletic fields, bike, and nature parks. As I push, I struggle to temper my assertive encouragement so that it doesn't morph into excessive pressure. Regrettably, I probably have gone too far on a few occasions even though I never tempt Phoenix to take physical risks beyond his natural abilities.

Navigating these sorts of risk-taking decisions is often more complex for the fathers whose children are living with a disability. The connection between risk taking and independence is especially salient for these fathers. Depending on their child's specific challenges, fathers sometimes find themselves wondering if they are asking their kids to do too much or not enough. How much should the father of an eleven-year-old daughter with cerebral palsy expect her to do for herself? Should a father of a blind seven-year-old daughter rearrange the house in significant ways to accommodate his child or should he make minimal, if any, accommodations to replicate for his child the type of environment she will face beyond the home? What about the father of a boy with Down syndrome who is now nineteen years of age—how much should he push the child to become more physically active by using food as a bargaining tool? How protective should a father be of his six-year-old son who has a connective tissue disorder? Should he limit the boy's siblings' involvement in formal sports activities because he wants to avoid hurting his son's feelings? Should he keep his son from playing outdoors? And when and how hard should a father push his seventeen-year-old quadriplegic son to learn to take charge of his bathroom regimen on his own? These are but a few of the dilemmas fathers face as they try to figure out a loving, effective fathering style that empowers their children to thrive to their fullest potential despite limitations that stem from their special needs.

On a more basic level, fathers and mothers can step forward to make decisions about the use of seat belts, helmets, and sunscreen as well as exposure to guns and video games. Overall, the fathers were quite firm about enforcing the use of seat belts and a little more lax but still fairly committed to encouraging their kids to wear helmets. Sometimes dads made exceptions about helmet use if the kids were just riding their bikes in the driveway or on a little traveled side road next to the house. Yet, for the most part, they bought into the philosophy that they should protect their children's brains. Not surprisingly to me—given my personal observations seeing fathers and their kids out riding their bikes—several dads admitted to not personally using a helmet when they rode even though they required their kids to wear one. This style of "do as I say, not as I do" has always puzzled me.

Over the past several decades the risk culture has changed dramatically. Many fathers grew up in an era where helmet use was not prevalent or was only beginning to take hold. As a kid, I never wore a helmet while riding a bike and I never wore a seat belt. Similarly, I never had a car seat for Scott or even used a seat belt for him when he was a toddler or young child. Moreover, when Scott was a young child he never saw me wear a seat belt. Much has changed in the thirty-one years that separate my sons' births. Phoenix has never seen me on my bike without a helmet and he's never seen me in a car without my seat belt buckled. Similarly, he has always been in a car or booster seat with the appropriate seat belt arrangements and he has worn a helmet while riding every day, beginning with his days on his tricycle.

Ironically, when writing this section I decided to rig a tire swing to one of my trees in the back yard for Phoenix, six years old at the time. He and I did this together and were both excited to test it out. It was only when I had him swinging so that his feet were about ten feet off the slopping ground that it dawned on me that I might want him to wear a helmet. A tree swing was new ground for me as a dad. "Will others think I am being an overprotective dad? Will they think I'm some sort of safety nerd?" I thought to myself. "Should it matter what others think? Of course not!" I let Phoenix swing without a helmet that first afternoon while monitoring him closely.

That day and the next, I tried but could not recall ever seeing a kid wearing a helmet while riding a tire swing. In my teenage world, I used a tree swing in the woods hung by some friends. We never thought to wear a helmet even though we did release moves at our relatively high-swinging apex. If our timing was good, we landed on an old, smelly mattress. If our timing was a little off, well, the hard ground reminded us to improve our timing on our next turn.

The following day Phoenix and I got situated to do another swinging session. I was revisited then by the description that Tivon gave me about cracking his skull when he fell off the monkey bars as a kid. The lingering headaches that have stayed with him throughout his life gave me pause. I immediately fetched Phoenix's biking helmet from the garage and he put it on without a second thought. He has worn it ever since and I've made his friends do the same when they're playing on the tire swing at our house. Times have changed.

Fortunately, I've never had to think seriously about whether I could afford to purchase safety equipment to protect Phoenix. And despite having little money when Scott lived with me in his early years, I had few worries about supplying Scott with a safe environment because I was a naïve young father and the cultural climate about childhood safety was far less intense.

Today, money, or the lack thereof, can affect how many dads make sense of risk culture and what they actually do to monitor their children's risk taking and protect them from harm. Even though dads often embrace their socially constructed roles of being the family and child protector, some are financially better equipped than others to act on their beliefs. Dads with few if any meaningful financial limitations can readily align themselves with their provider and protector roles by emphasizing the use of the newest and best safety equipment.[34] In contrast, low-income dads may struggle to find the discretionary income to purchase safety equipment for their children, or they may have to settle for items that are not as highly rated, or they may have to settle for previously used items. The price of helmets and car seats, for example, can quickly add up—especially if a father is supporting multiple children. Less affluent dads may also have to compromise on child care arrangements that place their children in situations where they are less likely to be watched carefully. More generally, unlike dads with money, those with limited incomes may feel they are unable to protect their children from various threats because they don't have the means to relocate their family to a new and presumably safer neighborhood and school environment.

Although money can sometimes make a difference, it's refreshing to learn from a large, longitudinal study in Japan that infants with fathers who are more active in caring for them when they are six months old (feeding, diaper changing, bathing, putting to sleep, playing, and taking for a walk) are less likely to incur unintentional injuries at eighteen months.[35] It's not clear why this pattern exists. However, the researchers suggest it could be because early paternal involvement is a proxy measure for the amount of supervisory time dads spend with their children as they develop, or fathers' involvement reduces mother's stress level and in the process enhances the quality of maternal care, or children who receive lots of attention from fathers may learn to behave in ways that are less sensation-seeking and risky. Another longitudinal study done in the United States shows that a positive father-child relationship may reduce the likelihood of injuries during middle childhood, especially for boys.[36] So there appears to be some evidence that fathers who are involved with their young children in supportive ways can help protect them from unintentional injuries.

SITUATED FATHERING

Being a dad doesn't occur in a vacuum—it happens in different types of places that may be more or less conducive for a dad to do certain things. In the past, my colleagues and I have written a lot about how various aspects of particular settings make a difference for how a father thinks about his child and interacts with the child in those places.[37]

When it comes to a child's health, a father's ability to encourage certain types of physical activities or healthy practices will be affected by features of his neighborhood and the larger community or city. If a dad has a field and pool right outside his back door and wooded trails for biking a minute away, it's a lot more convenient to direct a child toward good fitness habits than it is for the dad who lives in a rundown apartment building, in a neighborhood with extensive gang activity, and without outdoor recreational options nearby. Many kids live in subdivisions and neighborhoods devoid of these amenities and challenges, but they will be influenced by the distinct physical attributes of their surroundings (for example, availability of sidewalks and bike paths, level of traffic, yard size) and parental perceptions of how comfortable they feel allowing their children to navigate the space.

To think of fathering as being situated when it comes to health, fitness, and well-being issues means that circumstances associated with different sites and settings can influence how fathers orient themselves to their kids' physical, emotional, psychological, and spiritual health. *Chicagoland,* the CNN unscripted eight-part series that aired in 2014, provides a powerful reminder that many low-income parents living in Chicago, and many other places, keep their kids from playing outside because they fear that they will be hurt or killed by street violence. Recall too how Emmit's fears of a different type of unsafe neighborhood put a damper on his willingness to let his children play outside, especially without parental supervision.

Some fathers, like Joseph, are fortunate to live in neighborhoods where kids can freely play outside without worry. Because Joseph's yard is the biggest in the neighborhood, it has become the community hub for playing outside. Joseph is relieved that his four kids spend many hours at the house playing lacrosse, jumping skateboards, or swimming in the pool with the other ten or eleven neighborhood kids who show up at his house. He adds that "anytime somebody gets hurt, I'll see one of the kids coming in the front door . . . and they'll go back and they'll get the alcohol and peroxide and the gauze and the tissues and they'll come out there, and put a, bandage him up with Band-Aids or whether it's a roller bandage, they do a good job." Seeing his kids do first aid on their friends is particularly rewarding to Joseph because all of his children have taken the courses he's taught on CPR, first aid water safety, and first responding training for EMTs and paramedics.

For a different set of reasons, Chao, a thirty-eight-year-old Asian father of three kids, feels that he is much more at ease with his kids at home than when he takes them out in public because he has more control over his own setting. He feels it's "nerve-wracking" to be out at a soccer match for his daughter or at other activities because he tends to watch over his children like a hawk. His fathering style is partly tied to his concern for his son, who has a connective tissue disorder that places him in considerable danger if he gets bruised or cut.

While many fathers love doing activities that have health and fitness benefits with their kids on their property, many also enjoy creating special memories doing physical or health-related activities away from home. Some fathers spoke fondly of camping and hiking trips—sometimes in other countries, exploring new roads and trials on a bike, or being a coach for one of their kid's sports teams.

If we expand the lens of place to think of how well a community or city supports farmers' markets, co-ops, parks, and recreational facilities, including bike, running, and hiking trails, we can see more clearly how a father's options to be engaged in fitness activities with or without his children will be affected. In 2007, the American College of Sports Medicine (ACSM) developed a detailed American Fitness Index (AFI) that takes into account various aspects of how cities can affect the health of residents and mobilize community resources to enhance healthy lifestyles.[38] The composite index includes "personal health measures, preventative health behaviors, levels of chronic disease conditions, as well as environmental and community resources and policies that support physical activity."[39] A 2015 ACSM report assessed the fifty largest metropolitan areas in the United States and assigned the number one and two rankings to the Washington—Arlington-Alexandria (DC and Virginia) and Minneapolis–St. Paul–Bloomington (Minnesota) areas and the lowest rankings to Memphis, Tennessee, and Indianapolis-Anderson, Indiana.[40] Although the index does not incorporate information specific to men or fathers, it provides a general way to differentiate the community fitness levels for numerous major metropolitan areas. Thus, the average father residing in one of the highly ranked metropolitan areas should find it easier to adopt a healthy lifestyle than his counterpart living in Memphis or Indianapolis.

Similarly, a father living in a relatively small city like Boulder, Colorado, with its thousands of acres of recreational open space and nature preserves, is much better positioned to be a fitness-conscious dad than one living in almost any other relatively small city (that is one with about 100,000 people). In addition to the tangible parks, mountain trials, bike paths, and gyms, the collective spirit or consciousness of the people who live in a place like Boulder can encourage a father to pursue more joint physical activities with his kids. But even in leisure-friendly communities like Boulder some dads struggle to find the discretionary money and free time to invest in the recreational activities, equipment, and food choices that can promote their children's health and fitness.

Obviously, there are no guarantees that creating the recreational infrastructure will improve fathers and children's approach to health and fitness, but the path to adopting a healthy style of fathering will be more challenging without public support.

The lifestyle ideologies that permeate a place can matter a great deal for those who journey outside conventional patterns. Ronny, a thirty-nine-year-old father of two boys, currently lives in Portland, Oregon—an area that received the seventh highest ranking in the nation for its community fitness by the 2015 ACSM report. He feels that the places where he has lived have been rather progressive, so few people have felt at odds with him and his kids being either vegan or vegetarian. He feels that his kids have received a lot of support and the school system has been good about offering vegetarian meals for them. To his knowledge, the kids have not been teased at all.

Just as we can think about situated fathering, we might consider how men's fathering perspectives are influenced by the situated childhoods they experienced. As we've seen, growing up on a farm or near a wooded area is likely to influence the parenting values men bring to their own children. Similarly, being raised in a setting that has few recreational opportunities, no safe places for children to roam free of adult supervision, and no land for gardening can affect men's visions of what fathering entails. In general, various features common to rural, suburban, and urban living environments can all make a difference. Men's childhood experiences may, in subtle ways, continue to influence how they come to think about their own health, fitness, and well-being when they become adults and fathers.

4 ❧ TAKING STOCK AND ACHIEVING PERSONAL GROWTH

B<small>Y MOST ACCOUNTS</small> Owen has lived an atypical life. Now a fifty-three-year-old teacher, Owen understood early on that he was being groomed for the army. Much of what he did was designed to impress his father.

A well-traveled army brat, Owen was a precocious kid who was advanced four grade levels in middle school. He graduated high school at twelve and college at seventeen. During high school he was extremely small for his grade level and no longer competed in sports with his peers. Because his father pushed him, Owen learned karate and earned a black belt in judo, but he was not enthusiastic about either.

As a young man, he fulfilled his father's vision by joining the army. Throughout his many years of service as a combat engineer and paratrooper, he stayed fit as best he could for being one of the guys who got "thrown into the meat grinder." His more than two hundred jumps, extensive combat experience, and years of carrying heavy loads ravaged his body, and he left the service having endured two fractured hips, a fractured sacrum, a fractured vertebra, an impact fracture of his foot, a broken arm, multiple skull fractures, a broken jaw, a lacerated arm in hand-to-hand combat, and more. Beyond his physical injuries, Owen also suffers emotionally and psychologically from PTSD.

In retrospect, there's no telling precisely how, or to what extent, this troubling mix of conditions affected Owen's reentry into the civilian world. But they surely contributed to how his health and fitness declined from excessive eating and limited exercise. Dating back to his mid-thirties until he was forty-seven years old, Owen was in a downward spiral of gaining weight and becoming less mobile. He left the service weighing between 180 to 190 pounds and eventually ballooned to more than 340 on his five-foot, six-inch frame. For many years he used his kids as a physical extension of himself by asking them to do all sorts of things for him so that he would not have to get out of his chair or bed.

Then, in a chance meeting seven years ago, Owen says he encountered a man who fundamentally changed his life.

What he told me was that I was going to die and I kind of understood that. At an intellectual level, I had pretty much decided that I wasn't getting better, I was gaining too much weight, and I knew that my health was going to eventually fail me. But what he said to me was: "You are going to leave your wife without a husband and your kids without a dad. You are saying to them, every time you eat like this, . . . that you care more about eating than you care about being with them." And you see, being prepared to die is one thing. Yeah, I had come to this point where I had said, I am, there's no way I can work out, there's no way I can drop this weight, so I'm just gonna eventually just stay it out and die. But he made me realize that even though I was taking the easy way out, I was going to leave my kids in a bad place. And I hadn't really thought about that. So he reframed that argument for me and when he did that, it forced me to take action.

The very next day Owen did a strategic "pantry raid" and threw out a massive amount of unhealthy food. Once Owen nearly emptied his shelves he needed to come clean with his three teenage sons and wife about his new life vision.

The person who provided the "slap in the face" became Owen's yoga instructor. With his help, Owen lost 140 pounds within a year's time, 100 of which came off in the first six months. Now he eats vegan and weighs 160.

His sons were inspirational for him because he wanted to do things with them; he had missed out on quite a bit. Things were so bad that a preacher had taught his son how to ride a bike because he was unable to do so. True, Owen had to shift his thinking to overcome his lethargy and put in time and strenuous effort to transform his body, but his sons' support was also vital. His eldest son compiled a video of Owen's transformative experience and his middle son wrote a school paper about seeing his dad walk for the first time. The sons began to see their father in a whole new and positive light.

Although unique in its details, Owen's story is but one of many similarly intriguing tales that reveal how fathers navigate varied paths in the health matrix as boys and men. One way to look at the assorted stories is to consider how fathers' awareness of matters related to their own health evolves over time—before and after they have children. How do men's life experiences as men and fathers affect their distinct awareness of personal health and fitness and shape how they approach their children's health, fitness, and well-being?

PERSONAL HEALTH AWARENESS

Owen's story provides a glimpse of the myriad ways a man perceives his state of health and fitness over time. Initially, Owen showed himself to be a self-conscious youngster who was a tad insecure about his body because most of his classmates were so much older, bigger, and more mature. That awareness and self-image improved once Owen joined the army and distinguished himself as a capable soldier and judo competitor. With his departure from the army, Owen's mentality gradually evolved to the point where he resigned himself to being obese, unfit, and most likely destined to die prematurely. He eventually got to the point where he didn't spend much time thinking about his circumstances. And then his most recent shift in perspective— inspired by his future yoga instructor—primed him to remake his lifestyle and eating habits. Years later, in the midst of my interview with Owen via Skype, he pushed his chair aside to demonstrate his flexibility and balance. He did a one-legged standing yoga pose that culminated in his raising and fully extending his other leg against the side of his head. I was impressed. The stance was well beyond what I could do. Owen is now constantly aware of his identity as a rejuvenated, much healthier man.

Owen's life experiences also illustrate that there are many aspects to how a man thinks about his health, fitness, and well-being. To appreciate more fully how a man forms and expresses his identity in the health matrix, let's explore some overlapping questions.

Focus

How often and intensely does a man focus his mental and physical energies on his state of health and fitness? Does he wake up each morning well rested and immediately think about eating a healthy breakfast? Does he carefully plan his day so that he can eat well, work out, meditate, rehabilitate an injury, or do whatever else he might feel is necessary to stay in good health or regain his fitness? Does he seek out, read, and discuss materials on nutrition, fitness, and other topics related to self-care? Does a man with a debilitating health condition or an addict continually struggle for a period of days, months, or years trying to overcome a special need or an addiction that has defined his life? Or does this man fixate on his unhealthy condition and sulk?

Being conscious of his health status does not guarantee that a man is doing so in a constructive way. The mental activity can be directed toward managing a healthy life but it can also be spent idly on wishful thinking or mourning an out-of-shape, unhealthy existence.

In addition, personal reflections and actions in the health matrix can be in sync, but they sometimes are not. A man can think long and hard about his poor state of health, and he may even think plenty about what he should be doing to enhance his health and fitness, yet through choice or circumstance do nothing about it.

When fully engaged, he will be tuned in to his body, mind, and spirit. He will try deliberately to sustain or improve as best he can the quality of his health and fitness by monitoring what he eats; exercising regularly; seeing various health professionals as needed for checkups, screenings, and counseling; and eliminating poor health habits and unnecessary risk taking, such as his use of cigarettes, alcohol, drugs, or motorcycle riding, fast driving, and being in the sun without sunscreen.

Of course, men vary greatly in what they eat and what eating well means to them. I spoke to meat-eating fathers who believe a dinner is incomplete if meat isn't on the menu, as well as to fathers dedicated to either vegetarianism or veganism.[1] Although there aren't data to document how many men fit the former description, a 2012 Gallop poll found that only 4 percent of American adult men consider themselves to be vegetarians.[2] Most fathers live somewhere between these two extremes. Some pay attention to how much and what types of meat they eat.

Fathers sometimes acknowledge they are partial to certain ethnic or regional styles of cooking that are known to be high in fats, sugars, salts, or other unhealthy items. Their style of eating may be so normalized to them that they may seldom spend time consciously assessing how their diet is adversely affecting their health. And then there are the dads committed to staying away from fatty foods while noting their intent to eat lots of fruits and vegetables and avoid processed foods. They are more likely to incorporate their dietary decisions into their sense of who they are and what their health is like.

As we saw with Jeremy, vegetarian (and especially vegan) dads are often acutely aware of the ties between nutrition and health because of their unconventional eating practices. Compared to the typical meat-eating dad, they pay more attention to their food choices because they reject the American classics, including steak, hamburgers, hot dogs, meatloaf, pork chops, chicken wings, and fish sticks, to pursue alternative protein sources. Regardless of their choices, vegetarians and vegans are still exposed to the many threads of popular American culture, including the long reach of the Madison Avenue advertising machine that reinforces a meat-loving mentality.[3] Even though the motif of the "New Age man"—one who embraces his feminine side, supports women's rights, and rejects traditional macho posturing—has expanded perceptions of manliness in recent decades, meat consumption is still fiercely equated with a tough and hard masculinity in many social circles.

The television commercial Burger King aired in 2006 titled "Manthem" for the Texas Double Whopper illustrates how embedded the link between masculinity and meat-eating is in American culture. The opening jingle, "I am man, hear me roar in numbers too big to ignore, and I'm way too hungry to settle for chick food," is sung by a man headed to Burger King.[4]

He sings it to the melody of Helen Reddy's original song "I Am Woman," which highlighted women's empowerment in the 1970s. Today, the masses identify with the Burger King commercial, with its silly—not to be taken seriously—scenes of mobs of men doing "manly" things while eating a Double Whopper. The ad "works" because it captures the stereotype that eating meat reinforces men's manliness and empowerment.

More recently, in 2013, Taco Bell trumpeted its own appeal to a meat-eating emblem of masculinity by airing the Triple Stack Steak commercial depicting an unathletic-looking man sitting next to an outdoor court watching an intense game of pickup basketball with a voice-over presenting the man's critical commentary of the quality of the play. When the man puts down his steak sandwich and confidently walks toward the court, the voice-over initially directs a warning to the players on the court, "Bring your umbrellas, ladies, Hurricane Doug is going to make it rain." The message then ends by saying, "Three times the steak makes you feel like three times the man."[5]

In *Man vs. Food*, the popular food reality television series aired on the Travel Channel between 2008 and 2012,[6] Adam Richman, the series host, travels cross-country to experience the "big food" of various cities. An underlying and sometimes overt theme of these episodes is that men exude a beastlike presence and exert a type of "primitive masculinity" when they devour certain foods—especially meat.[7] With episode titles like "The Carnivore Chronicles" and the "Manimal," this show perpetuates images of how the typical man's consumption of meat furthers his standing as a "real" man.

One consequence of this cultural message trumpeting meat consumption as a symbol of manly behavior is that those who do not dine on meat are often directly and indirectly reminded that they have unconventional—presumably wimpy—food preferences.[8] They are often stigmatized and cast as having feminine personalities. Those reminders accentuate the unconventional eater's self-perceptions as a man who is oriented to a distinct vision of health and fitness and an alternative vision of masculinity.

Some men dedicate themselves to sustaining an exercise routine before and after having children. They tend to see their health-conscious disposition as part of who they are as men, but many also link their approach to being good fathers. Eating well, exercising, avoiding habits that have bad health outcomes, and generally being attentive to one's health is an important way a father can lead by example and show his love for his children.

Experiencing a serious injury or illness can leave the subset of dads who thrive on being physically active feeling disoriented and frustrated. A serious and painful degenerative disk problem incapacitated the previously fit and athletically inclined Joseph. He popped the strongest painkillers with no relief and rode electric wheelchairs at stores for the better part of a year before he opted to undergo surgery.

> I've never been out of shape until now and that's kind of hard on me. Because before I was encouraging and teaching the kids about physical fitness and strength training and everything with my boys and the whole time . . . I had a flat stomach and six-pack abs and I was working out every day. Now I've got a gut and I'm still trying to teach them right and I'm pretty sure they understand that I'm not able to be in the gym like I used to but I still feel like . . . I'm not maybe being looked at as much of a role model.

The surgery was a success. In time, Joseph recaptured his fitness level and now participates actively with his kids, but some dads are less fortunate. Physically fit fathers who develop diseases like MS and MD, become paralyzed, or lose limbs to disease, accidents, or military combat can sometimes adjust their personal goals and activities, but they tend to experience at least some frustration as men and fathers.

The addict who gets hooked prior to becoming a father as well as the addict who takes this self-destructive turn after having a child is set up to have serious moments of self-reflection about health and fitness. Whether men in either of these scenarios will actually "look in the mirror" is an open question. Being addicted to an unhealthy substance can inspire a father to mull over how his dependence and all that goes with it that keeps him from being a better father. All too often, though, an addict denies or rationalizes his circumstances and dismisses others' attempts to challenge his worthiness as a father. Therapy can sometimes help, but an addict has to be willing to seek out treatment and take it seriously.

Prior to spending time in prison and ending up homeless, thirty-two-year-old Austin spent two years as a stay-at-home dad caring for his two oldest kids, who were toddlers at the time. We initially talked about his addiction to cocaine and his use of other drugs, so I was not too surprised to learn that he often got high when he put the kids down for a nap. What did catch me off guard was his apparent defensiveness when I tried to clarify what he had been telling me about the timing of his drug use and caregiving for his children years ago. He needed it to be understood that the kids took a nap after lunch as a natural part of their daily routine. Austin would then get high and, according to him, the effect would largely be worn off by the time they woke. By his demeanor and tone, I sensed that it was important to him that I not think that he forced his kids to nap just so he could get high. The subtle distinction jibes with his intentions to rationalize that what he did— get high while he was in charge of watching his kids—was not all that bad.

Rudy, now a thirty-nine-year-old devoted father of four teenage daughters, had his own style of making sense of his methamphetamine and pot use during an eight-month stretch when he was a disgruntled stay-at-home-dad with two young children, including an infant. In retrospect, he acknowledges that his drug use ruined his life. However, during his "using" years he was largely oblivious to how his overall health and well-being were being jeopardized. Even today, he seems to minimize the effect his "very discreet" drug use around his children might have had on his ability to be a responsible father and interact with his child. "She was a baby and you can't really interact with an infant anyhow."

But caring for an infant is really serious business. Sonya, a nurse with many years of experience working in pediatric emergency medicine, knows all too well the dangers of mixing drug addiction with infant child care. She vividly shares a story about a married couple who had a five-year-old boy and a baby girl less than a year old. The incident that brought Sonya into contact with this family in the ER began at the family's house with the husband and boy napping while the mother was giving the baby a bath and preparing dinner. When the mother went to the kitchen to check on something in the oven she passed out. The father was awakened by the smoke alarm and found his son sleeping and his wife unconscious on the floor. He discovered the baby dead in the bathtub—she had drowned.

Although the couple and son were brought in to the ER to be tested for possible exposure to carbon monoxide, the results were negative, as Sonya had expected: the father was "very alert, kind of hyper vigilant" when he came to the hospital. Sonya witnessed the father confronting his wife: "She died, and it's your fault, she died!" Sonya reflects on her own response, "and to watch the grieving reaction of the little boy because I can still see him, too, he started crying and said, 'She didn't even get to have her first birthday.'" What struck Sonya was that the mother "never acknowledged any responsibility" and said it was an "accident" even though she had blacked out because she was addicted to painkillers. Sonya continues, "The father acknowledged that had they both not been addicted to pain pills that this wouldn't have happened." So, unlike Austin and Rudy, the father seemed to express a greater sense of accountability, although it took a horrific and very preventable accident to bring him to this personal realization.

Smoking. The substance addictions that receive the most public attention, and the ones that garner the most media coverage, tend to involve illegal drugs, such as crack, cocaine, heroin, ecstasy, speed, amphetamines, and marijuana. These drugs certainly touch the lives of countless fathers, children, and other family members; however, cigarette smoking is also highly addictive and can have dire consequences for long-term smokers. Tobacco use remains the single most preventable cause of death and disease in the United States. According to a 2014 Centers for Disease Control report, each year there are 480,000 premature deaths in the United States from tobacco use.[9] We also know that children are more likely to experiment with smoking and become regular users if their parents are smokers, so the consequences of fathers' smoking extend well beyond their own lungs and health. Children can also suffer by being exposed to secondhand smoke from their fathers. Even when pregnant women do not smoke, the secondhand smoke from fathers can pose a threat to the fetus and the mother's chances of experiencing postpartum depression.[10]

Since the early 1950s, advertisers have vigorously tried to associate smoking with displays of tough-guy masculinity. Most notably, from 1954 to 1999, Philip Morris used the iconic Marlboro Man in ads to target men with the intent of associating smoking with masculinity.[11] The figure was typically represented by a rugged-looking cowboy in a field with a cigarette in his mouth. Apparently the ads were successful: Marlboro became the best-selling cigarette brand in the world. But in the late 1990s, the Marlboro Man was shelved in response to the $206 billion Tobacco Master Settlement Agreement between the four largest United States tobacco companies and the attorney generals of forty-six states. However, the tough-guy angle linking smoking with masculinity was updated and recycled in 2013 by Blu e-cigarettes.[12]

Obviously, there is nothing masculine about dying prematurely from a preventable disease. Sadly, a former Marlboro Man who helped endorse cigarettes in the 1970s died in 2014 from chronic obstructive pulmonary disease (COPD), a disease primarily caused by cigarette smoking. Other actors who portrayed the Marlboro Man have also died of smoking-related illnesses such as emphysema and lung cancer. Ironically, the product that they represented for so many years eventually killed them.

Although the proportion of adult men who smoke has declined over the past fifty years, at least one in five men currently smoke. And as of 2010, a man's chance of being a current smoker was particularly high if he was living below the poverty level (33.2 percent) or had not earned a high school diploma (28.5 percent).[13] Unfortunately, smoking rates for the men in these two subgroups actually increased after 2005.

Many men who smoke are fathers. The dads who talked to me who smoke tend to recognize that it is an unhealthy habit and would be willing to quit, if quitting were easy. Most have tried one or more times to stop but have been unable to sustain their commitment. Some men who continue to smoke, as well as others who have given up their smoking habit, see how their identity as a father is connected to the message they have sent, are sending, or will send to their children.

Although the forty-year-old Frank talks about how he's been a good influence on his fifteen-year-old son's health habits, he tempers his assertion by noting that his son has seen him smoke. He's "pretty sure" his son doesn't smoke, yet he understands that his own behavior may play a role in the decisions his son makes. As Frank understands family life, "your parents are . . . the most important influence on our children so, more than not, the kids are gonna do what their parents do, it's just how it is. You know, it's how I believe it was with me. You know, both my parents smoked. I started when I was young. You know, they do what they see."

This type of potential influence from a father seems to matter to twenty-two-year-old Jensen as he thinks about his current smoking habit. He started smoking the day he turned eighteen, and, despite now having three kids, he has been smoking ever since. When he has the money, he smokes about two packs a day. Now that he is homeless and without a job, he only manages a half a pack or a pack. Although Jensen is not actively involved with his first two children, in part because of circumstances beyond his control, he professes that his mind-set and the circumstances with his one-month-old son are different. Becoming a father this time has "reopened my wanting to be healthy. . . . I don't smoke around him and really my goal right now is for me to not be smoking at all by the time he is old enough to remember anything."

Thoughts of being a responsible father certainly mattered to Troy the day he was stopped for a traffic violation years ago by a sheriff's deputy. After learning during the traffic stop that the officer had just been diagnosed with lung cancer, Troy quite smoking that day. "I feared for my child. Just because I like it doesn't mean it's worth it. I don't want to have it so when my wife and my daughters need me there, I can't be."

But having children has not stopped Grover from smoking. Instead, it complicates how he tries to makes sense of what being a good father entails. Now that he has been confronted with his teenage daughter's smoking, he sees firsthand how his unhealthy behavior is being passed down despite his warnings. The talks he has with his daughter are surely echoed throughout lots of households that include a parental smoker. Grover takes us inside his own family to share how he initially approached his daughter after he first caught her smoking marijuana that she had stolen from him and then suspected she was smoking cigarettes, too.

> "I know you grown and you don't want me to tell you what to do but I'm going to tell you them cigarettes will hurt you." She said "Well, Daddy, you do it." I said, "Yeah," I said, "that's why I'm telling you not to do it. You know what I'm saying? I say, don't do it. I'm telling you right now it's harmful." "Well, Daddy, I ain't gonna smoke but one cigarette." I said, "Yeah you might just smoke that one cigarette today, but if you like it, and something starts bothering you and worrying you, the first thing you're going to do is pick up another cigarette. And another one."

And that's exactly what happened. Grover's daughter is smoking a pack and a half a day and he continues to talk to her, trying to get her to stop. However, the authority of his voice on this matter is dampened because he has, in many ways, been a poor model of healthy behavior. Not surprisingly, his pleas have fallen on deaf ears. He has even bought her cigarettes on occasion, despite his conflicted views. Recently, though, he's starting to redefine what being a good father means as he reflects on how he enables his daughter's smoking habit. "Then it came to me, this is not the way to show a person that you care for them. Give them what you want, give them what they want gonna lead them to destruction or death. You know what I'm saying? That's just like conspiracy; you know what I'm saying. You know this here is going to kill them, why are you giving this to them? I've been praying about that."

Pepe, a sixty-six-year-old Cuban father with two kids, was a dad who smoked for thirty-three years before he quit after having a heart attack at age forty-eight and subsequently having bypass surgery. His children were sixteen and eight at the time. When asked why he hadn't stopped smoking when he became a father he falls back on the excuse about how difficult it is to quit. Pepe had integrated smoking into his lifestyle in order to man- age his work-related stress—a sentiment shared by other dads who smoke. Pepe doesn't credit his love for his children or even himself for overcoming his addiction. He believes it was because "there was a lot of people praying for me."

As I can attest to personally, a man's identity as a health-conscious per- son and his philosophy as a father can be affected by the image of smok- ing, even when he has never been a smoker. Part of my sense of health is that I would never want to ingest a substance that has been clearly shown to compromise lung functioning and make a person much more susceptible to getting cancer. As a child, I was around my mother a lot and she smoked regularly in my presence. This occurred in an era before the public was well versed on the negative effects of secondhand smoke. I quickly grew to dis- like the smell of cigarettes and decided I wanted no part of them. But, like many of the dads who have confided in me, I snuck a handful of cigarettes from her purse when I was twelve years old and smoked them down by the creek with a friend. Fortunately for me, that's as far as my smoking went because I didn't like the taste. Over the years since becoming a father, I've made a point of reminding my sons of my belief that smoking is a danger- ous, unhealthy habit. Both have embraced my message, one that is increas- ingly reinforced by public sentiment.

But Jay, a middle-class father of four, also thought his children were going to adopt his aversive attitude toward cigarettes. "Well, the smoking thing, I've pounded it into their heads from when they were born. That was always the big thing with me." As he begins to describe how smoking has entered into his experiences with each of his kids, his agitation is palpable. "The most disappointing thing is . . . every one of my kids either have at least, I know, tried smoking, and that was, horrific for me." Jay says it "tore me apart" when he learned that his eldest son was smoking. He was concerned about his health, but he also knew that his son knew how he felt about smoking. So Jay was offended that his son apparently didn't care enough about Jay's feelings to avoid it. His sentiments of feeling personally assaulted surface each time he learns that one of his kids has been smoking.

When Jay's son moved into his early twenties and found himself in the position of becoming a father himself, Jay recycled his message, saying, "You'd better stop." He added, "Now you're gonna find out what it's like. You don't want your kid to smoke and, he looks at you when you're smoking, how do you think, what do you think that's gonna do?" As far as Jay knows, something clicked, and Jay worries less now about that son smoking, but he's still concerned about his two younger children. Most recently, "I almost passed out. Never dreamt in a million years" was his reaction to hearing his teenage daughter answer yes to a doctor's question, "Do you ever smoke?"

Jay's stories about his children and smoking showcase his passionate antismoking stance. He's decidedly worked up after talking about his life-long distaste for his parents' smoking habits and his frustration with his kids' smoking escapades. As he winds down, he reasserts his inability to understand how his kids can smoke when they've seen their grandmother, his mother, die from lung cancer.

Managing a mind-set. Although some men drift into addictions and have a hard time recognizing their conditions, others are more like Jay—they are quick to guard against losing self-control by being dependent on a substance. Part of their mentality as a healthy person is that they must not succumb to needing a substance. That is Chad's view as a thirty-year-old who is trying to wean himself from coffee because he is concerned that he "couldn't get through the day without" it. Such dependency is inconsistent with his religious faith. "I don't want to have something in my life that controls me, like I have to have this, because I want to be free." Some of Eliot's stronger views about eating and other substances are reinforced by his commitment to the code of health that is central to Mormon culture. Based on the "word of wisdom," it stipulates that coffee, tea, alcohol, tobacco, and harmful drugs are off limits because they are addictive.

Clearly, some men and fathers give very little thought to their health and fitness. So what's up with them? In generations past, many fathers worked long hours at manual jobs or labored on their family farms. They didn't have the time or inclination to work out. They were doing physical work all day, sometimes seven days a week. Many already had an image of themselves as rugged, fit men who could handle doing a "real man's" work.

The fathers I interviewed sometimes described their own fathers and grandfathers in this manner. A few even adopted some version of this view for themselves. Steve describes his dad as someone who did strenuous work as a carpenter and had no interest in doing anything athletic for fun. Steve believes he's retained his father's traditional sentiment: he often chooses to do strenuous household jobs as a way to get some physical activity rather than avoiding them or paying someone else to do them. The essence of this mind-set is trying to work physical activity into one's daily life—à la the farmer lifestyle—rather than working out specifically. Steve, a white-collar professional, does much of the latter by playing tennis but incorporates some household chores into his scheme of physical activity as well.

The traditional mind-set linking manual labor to manly fitness is intimately connected to cultural values tied to social class standing and the types of work men do where they use their brawn and get their hands dirty for pay. I sense that many men who frame their worlds this way tend to devote little time or energy to thinking about their health and fitness. They simply go about living their lives knowing that they work hard at their jobs and are often very tired at the end of the day. That's how John, a forty-one-year-old father of two who unloads trucks for a living, evaluates his physical fitness. He acknowledges that he has a weight problem, but he thinks of himself as being in pretty decent shape because he has a physical job where he regularly picks up heavy materials for hours at a time.

Evaluating Personal Health

How does a man personally evaluate his condition? Is he extremely pleased, content, a bit concerned, or seriously worried? Someone can either focus on his overall sense of well-being or target more narrow areas of physical, emotional, mental, or spiritual health and possibly assess these areas differently.

A nearly century-old insight, commonly referred to by sociologists as the "Thomas theorem," is relevant here: "If men define situations as real, they are real in their consequences."[14] In other words, if men see themselves as being healthy and fit, they are likely to make choices for themselves and their children based on that perception. In some respects it doesn't matter that they (or their children) are actually unfit, even obese by conventional standards. The objective realities of, say, high levels of LDLs (low-density lipoproteins— bad cholesterol), high blood pressure (hypertension), and a poor body-fat ratio will increase a man's chances for negative health outcomes but they will not alter his immediate life choices if he is indifferent to them.

Self-relfection. Although I think of myself as being reasonably fit, I met fathers for this project who clearly were more invested in their health and fitness than I am. They had high expectations of what fitness represents. For example, Clive, a forty-five-year-old father of three preteens who has done twenty-six marathons and two full-distance triathlons,[15] assesses his current health and fitness this way: "I'm fit, not as fit as I want to be. I have an IRONMAN coming up in about a month and I went for a long bike ride yesterday and realized I'm not as fit as I want to be." This modest assessment comes from a man whose training runs are between sixty and ninety minutes and whose long bike rides on the weekend are three hours when he's preparing for a half-distance triathlon and four to five hours when he preps for a full-distance triathlon. His swimming sessions are forty-five minutes long a couple of times a week. Of course, Clive is using his own highly selective standard to judge himself; only a small percentage of men at any age, especially at forty-five, can roll out of bed tomorrow and do any of these activities, let alone all three sequentially on a race day.

A father of five, Giovanni regularly does endurance events like ultramarathons, sprint triathlons, Tough Mudder obstacle courses, and Go Ruck Challenges. Even though these events may fall short of the tenacity that was needed to do what Diana Nyad accomplished in early September 2013— swim 110 miles in open ocean water from Cuba to southern Florida—these events are not for the faint of heart or the poorly conditioned. Giovanni proudly states that he's often competing against men who were born twenty or thirty years after he was. A part-time life skills coach and physical trainer, Giovanni pays close attention to his eating habits and believes he has a remarkably healthy eating regimen. Having his children admire him for his fitness is an added benefit to the training and race events he does for "fun." He also values being able to show his children how resilient he has been in overcoming severe back problems and years of early childhood difficulties with his poorly developed legs.

On the mental front, Troy had a particularly difficult time when he thought about his three-year-old daughter during his time as a trauma nurse in Afghanistan in 2010 and 2011. Once he returned to the States, he was concerned that his wartime experience had negatively affected him. Among the many horrors of war he witnessed, Troy spoke vividly about touching and tugging on bodies that were piled on top of one another in a truck that had transported them from a bombing to his urgent care unit. When Troy returned stateside he increasingly had little or no patience for excuses. Seeing people in dire straits while overseas altered his perspective on his family's approach to life. He didn't want to hear his kids whining and complaining. To his credit, Troy demonstrated a proactive approach to fathering by making it a priority to see a therapist soon after he got back. He was sensitive to his mental health; he knew he was feeling mean and angry. His daughters picked up on his shift in temperament too so he sat down and talked to them about his deployment and his return home. Over time, Troy processed his wartime experiences and readjusted to family life as an engaged, nurturing father. "I found myself going back later on and trying to reverse some of the sternness that I laid on after I realized how different I was acting."

Some fathers, on the other hand, are not as proactive in seeking counseling after returning from overseas. Nick came back to the United States after several deployments to Iraq and Bosnia with a laundry list of serious ailments, including debilitating migraines, foot and knee injuries, ringing in the ears from a postconcussive blast, chronic back pain, and radiating leg pain. His back injury and migraines remind him constantly that he has life-altering physical problems that affect his self-perceptions about his fitness and his interactions with his infant son.

> Before that injury happened, I worked out every day. There were soldiers half my age that I could outrun them, outlift them, I could, out do anything with them. And now here I am two years later, and I'm afraid that if I pick [up] my baby that any time I could fall. I'm afraid, when I go down the stairs, I always

make sure I have one hand on a banister because I don't want to be the guy who falls down the steps with a baby in his hands. I'm afraid at times, I'm going to reach over and pick him up and I'm going to fall on him. Everything I do when it comes to him is calculated, so that I don't hurt him.

I sympathized with Nick's concerns about possibly hurting his baby because of his own frailty. Although Phoenix was bigger and less "breakable" at four and five years of age when I had my knee and back surgeries respectively, there were times with both injuries that I felt it unwise to place Phoenix on my back when I walked down the stairs from his playroom. Immediately prior to and after my first surgery I worried that my knee might give out and Phoenix and I would go tumbling down the stairs. Similarly, in the early days and weeks after my back surgery I was vigilant about not picking Phoenix up until I felt confident that we would both be safe. Postponing our playful, intimate "horsey-back" rituals was not easy for me. I felt as if something precious had been stolen, at least temporarily, from my son and me. Thus being a father accentuated my own self-consciousness about my less-than-desirable physical condition.

Personally, the most memorable moment in my interview with Nick was learning that I was the person he had talked to the most about his horrific deployment experiences. Although he shared lots of details with me, and got decidedly emotional while doing so, it seemed odd that the amount of sharing he did with me was more than he had done with anyone else. My initial perception of this was that it was unhealthy for Nick not to talk about his experiences to others. Yet he confidently asserts that he doesn't feel the need to discuss it and that he's privately dealing with it. His decision not to seek mental health counseling is a common response from men who have PTSD.[16] Despite his assertions, I have a hard time believing that any person would be unaffected by what he lived through and described for me.

Suicide bombers would constantly try to come at that gate and blow it up. . . . They would come with cars and vests, inevitably, they would blow themselves up and we would get a call saying hey, send someone down with a camera, or we need to take some pictures . . . inevitably when a suicide bomber puts a vest on . . . the bottom part of their body pretty much blows apart, and goes in different pieces in different directions, and their head because it's basically a big bone sort of shoots off and lands somewhere inevitably right side up, and everyone that I've seen, it always seems like the eyes are open and it's looking at you. So, usually, when I get to a scene, and I'll look for the head because I swear every time I see one, the head is looking at you. The one night I always remember is I got there and I looked and, I just remember the smell, and, and it was the guy's guts, and I looked over, and there it was sure enough, his head. One eye was opened; he was looking right at me. And I can remember, I remember distinctly, as vivid as . . . you and I look[ing] at each other, and I was telling the guy you know when I was at the VA they were asking me they go through this protocol of, there's six symptoms that determine if you have PTSD. One of them is do you vividly recall scenes from combat, and I'm like . . . I photographed it, so of course I remember everything about it. And then you go download it to your computer, and send it to somebody, to this person and that person.

Although Nick was not a father when he witnessed such human carnage, he became one soon thereafter. As his graphic descriptions led me to believe, the images he witnessed are still emblazoned in his mind. If Nick unknowingly is experiencing lingering psychological and emotional effects from his deployments, his son could indirectly be influenced as well.

I cannot say whether Nick is on the mark with his assessment that his psyche is fit. But I vividly recall participating in a psychodrama retreat many years ago and watching a former Vietnam vet open up for the first time about the emotional darkness he had buried for years. As a young man, one of his jobs was to load body bags of dead service members onto an aircraft. At the retreat, this stoic, rugged-looking man was by far the most reserved of the fifteen strangers who had assembled to share intimate details from their lives. He was there reluctantly, dragged by his fiancée, who apparently made his attendance a prerequisite for their marriage. On the final day, when it was his turn to have his session with the therapist encircled by the others, he broke down and wept as he unloaded his torment. Memories of that dramatic outpouring made me wonder if Nick was unaware of the deep mental and emotional trauma he harbors from experiencing wartime atrocities. Will that trauma, if it exists, affect the quality of his fathering long-term?

Servicemen like Owen, Nick, and the man I met at the retreat who return to civilian life after wartime deployment—especially those who have experienced wartime trauma—are at increased risk to encounter various mental health problems. The mental health issues veterans struggle with are often connected to a larger set of behavioral problems, including hazardous drinking, drug addiction, family reintegration issues, and incarceration.[17] The Veterans Administration, Wounded Warriors, and Paralyzed Veterans of America have organized diverse activities and treatment programs to help veterans' mental health and their transition back into their families. Although promising, these programs are still being evaluated. The research community does recognize that PTSD and other anxiety-related disorders can negatively affect family relationships for veterans who are fathers in the form of emotional isolation, substance abuse, domestic violence, and family dissolution. But much more is known about how these veterans struggle in their romantic relationships than with what happens in their relationships with their children.

The poor health of fathers returning from deployments is no trivial matter: large numbers of fathers and children have been affected since 9/11. More than 44 percent of active duty members have children, with a majority of those members being fathers.[18] Of the more than 1.2 million children with a parent who is an active duty member of the armed forces, 42.6 percent are children under five years of age.

Christal Presley, author of the powerful memoir, *Thirty Days with My Father*, is well aware of what it's like to grow up with a father suffering from PTSD.[19] Her father, Delmer Presley, was drafted before his nineteenth birthday and served a year in Vietnam. As a child Christal grew angry thinking that her father did not love her, when in reality it was PTSD taking over his mind. Delmar's PTSD surfaced when Christa was five and Delmer saw his friend's dead body in the highway after a car accident. This was a turning point for Delmar, who had not seen a dead body since Vietnam. For Christal, what ensued was a childhood full of unforgettable events and disappointment. Her dad would lock himself in his room for days at a time playing his guitar instead of playing with Christal. When loud noises struck, her dad would panic and go into soldier-at-war mode. Christal was embarrassed when they would eat at noisy restaurants. But even worse than this was when Delmer would take his shotgun to the nearby river, announcing to Christal and her mother that he was going to kill himself. As the years passed, Christal tried to find peace in other areas of her life, settling in another state and becoming an educator. However, she knew that she would never be at peace until she confronted her dad. When she finally faced her fears and approached him, it led to a series of intimate conversations over

thirty days. Ultimately, the book that emerged from these talks was thera-
peutic for her and has helped others who have loved ones suffering from
PTSD.

Incarcerated fathers and those who have been released represent another
important subset of fathers with significant health concerns. Compared to
deployed military fathers' experiences with returning home, incarcerated
fathers who reenter the civilian population and reengage with their young
children are likely to face an equally challenging, and sometimes more difficult set of circumstances. The public eye plays a role here because popular images of American soldiers returning from most overseas missions
stress their honorable service whereas public perceptions of ex-cons underscore the stigma associated with their circumstances.

In 2007, about 1.6 million children had a father in prison at midyear;
nearly half of those children had an African American father, many with
limited financial resources.[20] Many state inmates with children are in poor
health, and those problems are likely to persist when they return to civilian life. About 40 percent of incarcerated fathers indicate that they have a
current medical problem and 55 percent have some type of mental health
problem. At least 65 percent indicate they have an issue with substance
dependency or abuse. One reason these patterns are noteworthy is that
26 percent of fathers in the state prison system indicate that they provided
most of the daily care for their children immediately prior to their incarceration. Another 63 percent say they shared daily care for their kids. Fifty-
four percent report they were the primary financial provider for their minor
children before they went behind bars. Either directly or indirectly, the
problems incarcerated fathers experience can frequently have negative consequences for their children.

Making sense of personal changes. Although cultural forces clearly dissuade
American men from dealing effectively with injuries and illnesses, men's
reactions to physical and emotional problems tend to differ. Men are likely
to recognize on at least a superficial level that something is physically not
right with them, but they often completely dismiss it, don't take it seriously, or believe that they should just manage it in a "manly" way without
complaint or consultation.[21] With emotional difficulties, men may be ill
prepared to identify that something is even wrong. They may be oblivious to the symptoms or meaning of their unhealthy mood. Whether they

recognize they might have a problem or not, men are less likely than women to seek consultation for physical or mental health issues.[22]

When men do assess their health and fitness status they can use several different reference points for comparison. "The state of my health and fitness, relative to my age, is probably very good; relative to my needs and my desires, it's not very good," laments Cal, a fifty-nine-year-old dad of two teenagers. "I love being able to participate in every sport that I did when I was like, ten years old, but since I'm fifty-nine. . . . I've incurred a lot of injuries," he adds. Compared to other men his age Cal understands that he is in reasonably decent shape. But he has stubbornly held on to his youthful athletic vision of himself throughout the years. Doing so has created a dilemma for him because his mind and body are in a constant struggle as he tries to adjust mentally to his older, less reliable body. He remembers the times when he had more control over his body and could push himself to the max, not needing to fear that he might hurt himself. Looking back over the past two decades, as he makes more and more adjustments to accommodate his aging body he wonders "whether there is a threshold for me, where it's going to start to have a significant effect on my mental state of being." As he opens up, his words are laced with despair. "I truly feel a pain, in my stomach and, in my heart . . . and then I get past it, because I have to, and my level of disappointment lessens, but it is something that I've had a very difficult time with."

Michael Messner, a sociologist, has written about the difficulties many athletes have making the transition from being healthy, potent, and relevant to being "washed up," ineffective, and "old news."[23] Former athletes at various levels of competition sometimes struggle to re-create an identity that is not firmly anchored to their previous success in sports.[24] The transition can occur abruptly or gradually over time, but it often forces a man to see his body and his relationship to others in a new light. What about dads who are former athletes? What conditions determine how much they struggle as men and as fathers when their physical abilities fade? When do they successfully adjust and effectively shift their energies, resources, and dreams to their children?

Cal's mindfulness about the limits of his aging body and the mental gymnastics he's performed to accommodate his physical changes have become more complex since he had children. He believes he's been pretty good at sacrificing some of his personal health and fitness time over the years to care for his children. However, he struggles with what having athletic kids has meant to his psyche:

"Watching both of my kids, and especially my son, do things that I would love to be able to do, with him, or to just to do myself, because I can watch him do those things and still, there's a part of me that feels, 'Man, I can still do those things,' but I kind of know that I can't, at least to the extent that he does them, then it sort of makes it more difficult and more challenging for me to accept my place, as a fifty-nine year old, who's not building muscle but is maintaining what he has . . . that issue of mortality . . . comes into play, and that's difficult for me, but, I'm doing it, but it's no fun."

Control

To what extent does a man believe he has control over the circumstances that influence his state of health and fitness? When a man identifies particular circumstances as ones he believes he can control he may think about himself differently than when he believes he doesn't have much, if any, control over the forces that affect his health. Things are not so straightforward though, because different men may perceive the same circumstances as being controllable or uncontrollable. A man who is mindful of his health and committed to being fit may be motivated to see various conditions as under his control. For example, compared to the dad who is more lackadaisical, a health-conscious dad may be more likely to quit a demanding job, submit to a difficult addiction recovery program, or eliminate other leisure activities to squeeze in exercise time early in the morning or late at night.

Those battling a debilitating illness like MS, Parkinson's disease, heart disease, or those who are severely visually impaired may feel constrained in what they can do to maintain or regain their health or even be physically active with their children. I suspect most fathers take for granted how critical their eyesight is to how they think about themselves as fathers. As fathers we see and respond to our children's smiles and frowns, celebrations and tantrums, and all manner of physical expressions that mark their lives. By literally seeing our children we are able to assess what they need and want as well as what they think of us. We clearly see what they are eating and how much they're eating as we sit down with them for a meal. We register how their physical bodies change as they mature from baby to teen to young adult and we look on with curiosity and sometimes disbelief when they adopt new hair styles, forms of dress, piercings, and body ink. We also use our sight to teach our kids skills associated with physical play and sports—throwing, kicking, and catching a ball; riding a bike; running and jumping; swimming; and doing calisthenics. But dads who are blind must adapt to fathering their children without being able to see them.

Living with diabetes since he was four, Morris suddenly lost sight in his left eye because of glaucoma when he was about twenty-three. Four years later, after he had become a married stepfather to an eight-year-old girl and six-year-old boy, he underwent what was to be routine cataract surgery on his right eye. When he awoke from the procedure he unexpectedly began the first day of his life as a stepfather who was completely blind. Despite this setback, Morris has been actively involved in the kids' lives by going to their pediatric appointments, talking to them regularly about nutrition, and showing them the value of having a healthy diet. In addition, he believes his religious commitments have strengthened their mental fitness. In turn, the kids have become attentive to his new needs as a man who cannot see, and they are very protective of him. Morris shares with me that the girl is sensitive to his moods and helps pick up his spirits when he's sad. The boy wants to walk him everywhere. Both kids integrate Morris into family games like Wii bowling, and they narrate movies for him. They are proud of his accomplishments, including his being able to walk by himself to the bus stop. Each enjoys introducing their friends to him. However, aside from taking walks with them, Morris is no longer able to be physically active with them doing such things as riding bikes or playing catch.

Compared to Morris, Campbell had more time to adjust to losing his vision. The retinal disease that was diagnosed when he was thirty eventually forced him to surrender his driver's license by fifty and has left him with no functional sight at age fifty-seven. Campbell was forty-two when his son was born, so he had plenty of years to bond and be physically active with him before he lost his vision. To this day, Campbell works out regularly and was training for a seven-day, five-hundred-mile tandem bike ride with a friend when we talked. He and his teenage son sometimes work out together at the gym lifting weights and exercising on adjacent stationary bikes or Stairmasters. They also do sit-ups and squats at the house. Campbell claims that being a father has encouraged him to be more fit and to show his son that he can overcome anything. In his mind, actions are his main teaching skill.

I was impressed to hear how supportive Morris's and Campbell's children have been as the men have made adjustments in their lives to make the best of their circumstances. The kids' actions, and the meaning they have for these two men, illustrate how fathers and children can jointly react to one another's health needs.

Social Networks

How does a man perceive that family, friends, and colleagues affect his personal approach to health and fitness? Is he able to develop the kinds of partnerships that enable him to promote his own and his children's well-being? Does he find himself surrounded by health-conscious and physically active family members and friends, or is his intimate circle largely made up of inactive people who eat poorly and use harmful substances? Are family members directly supportive or dismissive of his efforts to be health-conscious? Family also can come into play indirectly if a father is committed to remaining healthy because he wants to be involved in his children's and grandchildren's lives, or be there for his romantic partner for years and years to come.

Campbell was full of disdain for his father, who he felt did a poor job of loving and nurturing him, so he was fully committed to giving his son a different sort of experience. By being "all in" as a father, Campbell learned to deal indirectly with physical adversity because his son has lived with diabetes since he was two. A former army officer, Campbell is compelled to lead by example. He wants to demonstrate to his son his independence and ability to overcome the challenges he faces as a visually impaired person.

But Campbell's experience with his son is not a simple one-way relationship. They have developed a strong bond of mutual trust as they've learned to help and depend on each other. As a man who is now legally blind, Campbell appreciates deeply how he has increasingly grown to trust his son. A year before we met, Campbell was on vacation in West Virginia with his son and they journeyed, at Campbell's request, into a cavern that was 167 feet below the surface. As Campbell recalls, once they walked down the stairs they entered a space that was "pitch black," with "slippery paths," and "cliffs everywhere." Campbell's reaction was immediate and intense. He told his son, "I'm insane for being here. I can't see and I'm gonna get killed." Campbell explains to me, "It's like 50 degrees under the ground, I was sweating, trembling, and I was freakin' out." Yet his son was not prepared to leave. He squeezed his father's hand and said, "Look, you said this is trust, God put us here for a reason, you have to trust. Do you trust me?" When Campbell said he did, the boy replied, "Let's do this." The gesture and words relaxed Campbell who went on to finish their exploration ninety minutes later with his son narrating in vivid detail what the cavern looked like. Campbell and his son's mutually supportive relationship illustrates one version of how reciprocity can be expressed in the health matrix—one parent and one child each depend on the other to deal with their respective special needs.

Family support can be vital in more typical settings too. "We're a pretty health-conscious family," says Rudy as he illustrates how his awareness for his health and fitness is intimately tied to family conversations and rituals that include his teenage daughters.

> We all have watched so many documentaries on health food and food and slaughterhouses and all that, and I have all girls, that are all you know, beautiful and sort of vain, and so health is very important, we're always bent toward proper nutrition and healthy eating, although we like our macaroni and cheese sometimes too, but we try to avoid processed foods completely, we try to eat about 80 percent vegetarian and most of the meats we eat are chicken, so a little bit of pork and a little bit of beef sprinkled in there.

As they banter, Rudy and the females in his household look out for one another and hold each other accountable for healthy eating habits. For instance, they tell each other how many days they've gone without eating meat or processed food. "We keep track individually, like it's something personal for each of us." Slipping into his fatherly voice he mimics how he talks to his athletic daughters. "Are you drinking water? What do you got in your lunch? You got a banana, you got some apples, what have you got? Where's your nutrition coming from? All that ain't good enough, let me get you this drink." Although Rudy's questions are designed to ensure that his daughters make sound nutritional choices, the exchanges reinforce Rudy's personal conviction to eat well too.

Along with his daughters, Rudy's wife is very much an active player in the family health matrix. When Rudy and I spoke he was excited to start a three-month nutrition and fitness program his wife ordered that would be arriving by mail later that week. Rudy and his wife planned to do the program with their daughters in the mornings.

Although men today are more likely to take the initiative and attend to their own health needs, the reality is that many partners and mothers, like Rudy's wife, still play a critical role getting the men in their lives to be more attentive to their health and fitness.[25] I saw this firsthand throughout my life as my mother monitored my father's eating habits, encouraged him to seek medical consultations, and faithfully made sure he took his many medications as directed.

Becoming a family man, especially in more recent years, has fueled Rudy's motivation to pay attention to his health and fitness. As he thinks about living family members and those yet to be born, his sentiments echo those of many fathers I interviewed. "I want to live longer than I ever wanted to live [before] so I can have an impact and be a part of them as long as I can. And I want to be there for my wife too, for sure, I don't think, I don't want to leave her alone. . . . I want my grandkids to get to know who I am, I want to be able to share my story personally with them . . . [I want them] when they're at that place in their life to be able to close their eyes and remember what grandpa said."

Rudy uses his dreams of being an engaged grandpa as shorthand to depict his frustration that no one in his family paid close enough attention to how the doctor dealt with his high school football knee injury. Looking back, he is disappointed that no objections were raised when a teenager was given 250 Percocets that lead to his addiction problems In his mind, his family didn't try to understand the "psychological damage" he experienced from "losing everything and all my hopes and dreams" because his injury ripped away his major college scholarship opportunities. As Rudy notes, unlike his parents who didn't talk about personal issues with him or other family members, "I talk about everything; I just want to share; I want to have longevity in my life." If he gets his wish, his longevity will be secured in the minds and hearts of his children and future grandchildren because he has been more attentive to their needs and has shared his years of wisdom with them—something his father did not do.

With passing generations, public sentiment seems to be that parents and children living in contemporary families are more likely to talk to each other about sensitive topics like sex, contraception, sexual orientation,

STDs, drugs, eating disorders, and special needs as well as more basic topics such as nutrition and exercise, all of which have implications for health
and fitness. Public health professionals have been eager to promote parent-
child discussions about health-relevant matters. Reports on the effectiveness of the Parents Speak Up National Campaign (PSUNC), sponsored
by the U.S. Department of Health and Human Services, indicate that this
initiative encourages mother-child communication about sex.[26] It is not
particularly effective in promoting fathers' communication with their
children, however.

The image of dad or mom as a friend is probably increasingly common
among recent generations of children and young people. Many of these
kids have navigated major portions of their lives with parents living apart.
They have witnessed their parents dating, living with, and marrying individuals who are not their biological parents. So, too, growing numbers of dads
are adopting a more nurturing, expressive style of fathering that is likely to
open up communication channels between them and their kids.

We live in a world where parents and their kids have packed schedules,
less time for shared meals and real face time, and parents are less likely to
live with their kids full-time for years of their lives. So I wonder whether
recent cohorts of dads are actually talking to their kids about health and fitness issues more than earlier generations of dads. If I base my impression on
the talks I've had with my limited sample of fathers, then my answer is yes—
dads are more aware of health issues and are having more health-relevant
talks with their kids. A case in point involves the fairly recent surge in attention being given to sports activity and concussions. Sonya, the pediatric ER
nurse, independently confirmed my suspicion, based on her twenty years of
experience, that contemporary fathers seem more mindful of head trauma
and concussion issues when she's interacted with them and their children in
a hospital setting. Over time more fathers have moved away from their old
school approach of matter-of-factly telling their kids to shake it off and have
instead become more comforting with their kids who have had significant
hits to the head.

Today, parents and their kids who are old enough to peruse the Internet have unprecedented amounts of information readily available to better understand health-related issues. Although the content found online is
sometimes unreliable, fathers and their children can use this information

to focus attention on some aspect of health, fitness, or overall sense of well-being. In doing so, they can also reinforce or alter their self-image of being a health-conscious person.

After a father told me about Fooducate, the phone app that helps its user assess the healthiness of food items, I began in June 2013 to use it in grocery stores with Phoenix. On our first day we scanned two different types of shredded wheat cereal new to us, our favorite burritos, and a low-fat lentil soup I consume regularly. We had a telling exchange when he approached me with big eyes and a box of honey shredded wheat cereal to purchase. Without looking at the label I balked immediately, assuming it was too sugary. But I complied with his request that I scan it. When, much to my surprise, the grade "B" appeared on the screen, he quickly and confidently reminded me, with a sly smile this time, that my lentil soup had also received a B rating. I caved in to the little negotiator and allowed him to put his cereal into our cart. From that day forward this item became part of our regular rotation of cereals. After our inaugural use of Fooducate we immediately incorporated it into our ritual to determine the quality of our preferred food choices. By using it for the past three years, we have both grown more mindful of and talkative about what we eat. It has also given me an objective means to filter my disapproval and buffer his discomfort with hearing no directly from me.

Family Health Legacy

Is a man's personal health awareness connected to some type of family health legacy? For example, is he intimately aware that his father or other relatives suffered from particular types of ailments that tend to have a genetic component such as high blood pressure (hypertension), diabetes, and cancer?

Seeing himself as part of a genetic family tree that has been rendered vulnerable by disease can heighten a man's awareness about his own health and fitness. He may become more sensitive to his body if he believes he needs to be extra vigilant about his and his children's health because they are predisposed to unhealthy outcomes. The health matrix idea showcases how the dad thinks about his family elders' health problems and then adapts his lifestyle accordingly. One way he may adapt is by encouraging his own child to notice that the grandparents or aunts and uncles are struggling or have died from specific ailments. Several fathers I encountered embrace the idea that they need to educate their children about their relatives' health. Although this perception is strongest when fathers are concerned about their own family's health history, some may be even more vigilant if they believe the health history on the mother's side is poor as well.

At fifty-nine, Zeke is quite concerned about his family health history, which includes his father dying of heart disease at age sixty-one. His worries may be well founded: he has had a series of heart problems and was diagnosed with diabetes five years ago. It was then that he enrolled his kids in a research study that tracks aspects of their blood over time to explore intergenerational genetic connections. Zeke has been very open with his kids about his father's and his own health problems.

Gerald, another father who is conscious of his family genetic health profile, has not gone for a physical in fifteen or twenty years even though he works in the medical field and has good health insurance. He doesn't even know if he's healthy, nor does he have a workout routine beyond doing pushups. Gerald joked about his philosophy—"As long as I'm walking and I'm talking, I feel like I'm O.K." The day we talked, he claimed that he was going to make a doctor's appointment the next day, although I have my suspicions that he didn't. Unlike his parents, who didn't talk to him about his unhealthy family medical history, he has shared that information with his teenage son. Ironically, he acknowledges that he is genetically predisposed to experience negative health outcomes, but he doesn't seem too concerned about his health.

My own dad was first diagnosed with vascular dementia in the early 2000s when he was in his late seventies. In some ways his experience has become part of my own perception of a family health legacy. I wonder from time to time if any of my forgetfulness might be a precursor to the more serious types of difficulties Dad experienced. While I joke about it, I sometimes reflect on what it might mean that Phoenix at the age of four and five was dominating me in our memory game matches using *Toy Story 3*, *Spider-man & Friends*, and *Fantastic Four* characters. To make matters worse, he has often won handily without even paying close attention!

I realize my health profile currently doesn't include the risk factors that increase a person's chances of developing dementia. Nonetheless, it registers with me that some of the diseases that cause dementia can be inherited, and that persons with a particular genetic makeup are at a higher risk to develop dementia.[27] Being a later-life father for Phoenix, I occasionally think about what it would be like to confront dementia's debilitating effects and be less engaged with Phoenix when he's still a young man.

Whether it is dementia, cancer, MS, alcoholism, or some other health condition, advances in biomedical technology are likely to make it easier for fathers with reasonable access to the health care system to learn more about their DNA-based family medical history. As men learn more about their personal risks for contracting certain diseases they may be compelled to alter how they think about themselves as men as well as fathers.

Perceptions about inherited genes and the family healthy legacy more generally also have a bright side for some fathers, me included. As I wrote in chapter 1, despite their relatively poor health and bad fitness habits, my grandfather and father significantly outlived their contemporaries. Thus, when I look forward to my own life span I anticipate that my genes are likely to serve me and my offspring well.

Sources of Motivation

What specific conditions motivate a man to develop a keener self-awareness about his health status? Clearly, lots of circumstances can affect how self-aware a man is in his daily life about his health and fitness. Rudy, Zeke, and Gerald's stories emphasize how aspects of a man's social network and family health history can make a difference. In addition, on an individual level, features of a man's work can increase his body awareness and motivation to be fit.

Terry, the very athletic father we met in chapter 2, has sustained his fitness and good health throughout his life, in part because he has always possessed a fitness mentality. But he is also one of the many fathers who became self-aware in another way once his children entered his life. Terry begins, "It's important to keep my health because I want to be around for them, and that's the thing I think of the most." His commitments to his own and his children's health receive an extra dose of reality because he's a nurse and health care educator. In his work he sees "people come in with deteriorating health and MIs [myocardial infarction, or heart attack] and type 2 diabetes and hypertension and all of the complications that go along with all of those things at such a young age. . . . That's why I continue to drag my butt into the gym and that's why I continue to go for walks and just do everything that I can."

One would think, then, that dads like Terry who have jobs related to health care or who work in the fitness sector would be well positioned to have the book knowledge and the professional life moments to prepare them to be more attentive to their own health, and, ideally, their children's health. I definitely talked to men who fit that description. As a personal trainer, Giovanni has been well positioned to pay close attention to his health and fitness while he coached and mentored his own kids to invest time and energy into their bodies when they played and trained for sports and when they made food choices.

Yet I also became good friends with a young doctor almost twenty-five years ago who exemplifies the other side of this pattern. I was surprised by his poor eating habits and limited investment in exercise. He usually skipped breakfast, and his lunch often consisted of a candy bar. Even his more wholesome dinners were often eaten late at night. He played soccer less than once a week and that was essentially his only planned exercise. Ten years later, having fathered two children by then, he ate much the same diet, and now had no time for or interest in playing soccer.

The high stress and demanding hours for many in the medical field can make it difficult to find the time and energy to engage in a regular exercise routine, get a reasonable amount of sleep, and eat reasonably well. So too the unhealthy food environments at hospitals, physicians' offices, and conferences contribute to physicians' poor eating habits. Lenard Lesser and his colleagues argue in a compelling essay in *JAMA*, the American Medical Association's flagship journal, that medical institutions should be more proactive in fostering a healthy food policy for all sorts of events.[28] They challenge doctors and the medical institutions they represent to take the lead in promoting better eating habits for the general public just as they helped reduce smoking trends decades ago.

Research that actually looks at health care professionals' own health and fitness has produced a somewhat mixed picture. The popular cultural image of the "unhealthy doctor" appears to be part fact, part fiction.[29] On the mental health front, a number of studies of physicians in the United States and other Western countries reveal that physicians, especially young doctors, have high rates of depression, anxiety, burnout, addiction to alcohol and drugs, and misuse of prescription drugs. In some studies their rates exceed those of the general population. In particular, physicians are five times more likely than the general public to misuse prescription drugs (for example, benzodiazepines and opioids).[30] And while male doctors on average live longer than their nonphysician counterparts, controlling for social class differences, and doctors tend to die from the same causes as the general population of men, physicians do have higher suicide rates.[31] One research team that studied mortality rates among physicians in the United States concludes that "considerable evidence" supports the claim that "individuals who have received medical training make healthier choices and therefore have lower mortality rates."[32]

Yet physicians collectively have considerable room for improvement if they want to be seen as ideal models of health and fitness. The 2004 Physicians' Health Study reveals that 44 percent of physicians are overweight or obese.[33] A later study of 763 physicians in California (75 percent were male and roughly 78 percent had children) finds that 53 percent self-report severe to moderate stress, 35 percent indicate that they never or only occasionally exercise, 27 percent say they either never or only occasionally ate breakfast, 21 percent work more than 60 hours per week, 13 percent are using sedatives or tranquilizers, and 7 percent are clinically depressed.[34] Whether doctors with kids treat themselves any better than those who are not parents is an open question.

The professional world of health and fitness is quite broad. It includes not just those involved in medicine but individuals trained as physical therapists, occupational therapists, personal trainers, and nutritionists. Although studies haven't systematically looked at the health status of these nonmedical professionals in the same way doctors have been studied, I suspect they tend to pay more attention to their own diet and exercise routines than the typical dad. They may also be more focused on these areas for their own children. With one notable exception, this pattern seems to hold true for the handful of dads I interviewed who had these sorts of careers.

Lewis, a forty-nine-year-old personal trainer who has been avidly lifting weights since his mother bought him a weight set when he was twelve, is committed to fitness and healthy eating. Through hard work, determination, and his mother's early support he transformed his identity as an overweight kid who topped out at 285 pounds as a five-foot, eleven-inch teenager. He now takes great pride in how he looks and feels. As a father of a twenty-year-old daughter who lives out-of-state and two stepchildren who live with him, Lewis reaches out to his kids by adapting the approach he uses to assess his clients' needs. He champions the "no one size fits all" approach, recognizing that there are different ways to reach young people and encourage them to be accountable for their own health and fitness. "You are your own manager" is the motto Lewis lives by and tries to pass on to his clients and children.

Changing Health Status

Finally, to what extent does a man see his condition as being in a state of flux—for better or worse? Different men may have a similar view of the quality of their current health and fitness status, but one may be more optimistic that he's improving than the other, who may be concerned that his health is on a steady or rapid decline.

The same forces that inspire fathers to become more cognizant of their own quality of health and fitness can lead men to believe that their health is changing. In some instances fathers are inspired by their children's increased attention to diet and exercise. They jump on the health and fitness bandwagon and get more serious about their eating habits and physical activity.

Getting positive feedback from family and friends can also be an added incentive for fathers to sustain their efforts to adopt healthy habits. One man talked about having a toddler son say that his "belly was getting smaller," which made it easier for him to keep on dieting. Another child was there for his dad during a two-week period when the dad, who had been a habitual smoker for many years, was able to quit. With watery eyes, the forty-one-year-old John recalls how his son "was on me every day. Always giving me props. 'Dad you're doing good! Dad, I'm proud of ya.'" Unfortunately, John picked up smoking again after a few weeks even though he freely acknowledges his son's warnings to him are well founded, and he struggles knowing that he is disappointing him. In John's case, despite his inability to respond well to his son's pleas—effectively locking himself into a limbo state in which the prospect of becoming a nonsmoker is only a remote dream—he is at least more conscious of his health dilemma. That consciousness is an important first step to changing bad habits.

CONNECTING PERSONAL HEALTH
AND CHILD WELL-BEING

As we've seen, some dads are motivated to pay attention to their own health and fitness because they want to pass down to their children useful information and a life perspective about staying healthy. When I ask dads to take stock of what they have done well to promote their child's health they sometimes speak about how they use positive and negative personal life experiences to teach their kids lessons.

Two basic ways a father can teach his children are to lead by example and to try to instill the values that are central to his life perspective, or to reveal his past or even current lifestyle warts and encourage his kids to make very different choices than he did. Sometimes a father who has had a turning point experience and has become much more health conscious may adapt both strategies. How a father is able to communicate successfully to his child using either of these approaches obviously depends on the child's developmental stage and personal interests. The father's own priorities, state of mind, and health status come into play as well.

In Terry we have a prime example of a man who lives his own convictions to express a caregiving style of fathering. Terry has "preached" and demonstrated health and fitness lessons to his biological children and stepchildren ever since they came into his life. He talks extensively to all his kids about nutrition, sleep, and exercise. Terry feels good about the influence he's had on his kids; he's taught them to be self-motivated about taking care of their minds, bodies, and spirits.

This type of adult caregiving—referred to in academic circles as "generativity," was first introduced by the famed psychologist Eric Erikson decades ago.[35] In its broadest sense, a generative spirit refers to efforts "to pass on valued traditions, to teach key skills and viewpoints, to communicate wisdom, and to help younger generations reach their full potential."[36]

I learned part of Terry's generative story about ten years ago when I first interviewed him for a book I was writing about stepdads. More recently, when I turned my attention to understanding the father-child relationship in the health matrix I immediately arranged to talk to Terry to get an update on his life as a father. My impressions were confirmed: Terry remains committed to leading by example in what he eats, how he exercises, how he tries to avoid risky behavior, and how he tries to have a spiritual presence in his children's lives. It came as no surprise that the kids who were in his life before and the stepkids who have come into it since have all responded at least reasonably well to his message.

Can a dad with poor health habits engage in generativity by telling his kid to "do as I say, not as I do?" Perhaps. But a child will most likely process the message as less authentic and in turn resist it.

I found it curious that fathers were more likely to talk about watching what they ate to set a good example rather than making a similar point as someone who exercised regularly. Maybe children process parental messages about diet, risk-taking behavior, and fitness differently. If they do, fathers might be able to get away with asking their kids to practice what they preach.

"That was a pretty consuming sense of who I was," Marshall replies as he explains how being overweight as a kid affected his identity growing up. Although his self-image has improved somewhat over the years, this thirty-three-year-old stay-at-home dad of a three-year-old son and one-year-old daughter still struggles to get past the lazy moments in his life. He says that he has given his wife the green light to harp on his eating and exercise habits because he doesn't want to be a "bad example" for his kids.

Overall, he believes he has done a good job of promoting a broad eating experience for the kids. He has also tried to show them that being active is fun. Yet Marshall would like to be a better role model for being active. He believes he's still learning to take care of himself and he wants to instill values about health in the kids so that it becomes second nature for them to make healthy choices when they get older. His goal is to provide them with the support he didn't have. Marshall also doesn't want his kids to have to experience a "come to Jesus sensation" of realizing that they need to take better care of themselves, as he did when he went to college. Embarrassed, Marshall recalls his "tipping point" from his college days. "I woke up in the ER with staples in my head because either I had fallen or I had been mugged or something, I still don't remember what happened." All he could tell his mother who was sitting next to him was that he was drinking at a party.

After doing a stint in the army reserves he found a more productive path as an adult and has a better grip on his personal health issues. He currently is exploring ways to manage the self-esteem problems that stem from the poor self-image he developed as an overweight child. Joining Weight

Watchers and losing some pounds was a concrete step in that direction. He incorporates his kids into his personal quest by telling them, "Daddy is trying to eat healthy and stay fit." Marshall's kids are now paying attention to him when he pulls out his weights. Sometimes they try to participate, and his three-year-old son even suggests they do yoga exercises together.

Marshall's story highlights how a lifetime of struggles with health and fitness can motivate a man to turn things around to ensure that his children develop a healthier perspective. But the health matrix for some fathers is much more complicated, especially for fathers whose children have chronic health conditions and special needs. These circumstances can put fathers' caregiving perspectives and skills to the test whether the fathers are healthy or not.

5 ❧ CHRONIC CHALLENGES

W<small>HEN</small> P<small>AUL HAD BREAKFAST</small> with his fourteen-year-old son, Philip, and the rest of the Boy Scout troop one sunny January morning in 2009, he had no idea his life was about to change so drastically. After breakfast he helped the guys for a couple hours make minor adjustments to their mountain bikes. The boys were eager to explore some of the wooded trails of Florida.

Several other dads accompanied the boys on the ride while Paul stayed at camp to work on a newsletter for his business. An hour or so later, immersed in his writing and formatting, Paul was interrupted by a call from one of the dads on the ride. Philip had taken a spill and his "face was cut up kind of bad." The dad encouraged Paul to head out immediately to their location. On the way Paul mulled over how he planned to deal with the situation; he and his wife had decided that if a health concern arose for them that they would not get admitted to a hospital. They did not have health insurance; they simply couldn't afford it.

In a deliberate voice, this longtime scoutmaster with extensive first aid training and previous experience as an x-ray tech relives the moment he arrived next to Philip lying on his back in the dirt. "At that point, I mean he was cut up and stuff in the face, but I mean I've seen horrible stuff come through x-ray so . . . that didn't bother me too much. I can get over that kind of stuff. He couldn't feel his legs and that was bad, but I kind of go into, I mean I've done so much emergency work anyway that I kind of go into a mode where you get the job done and worry about the rest of it later."

Philip, a big kid who weighed about 215 pounds at the time of the accident, had switched bikes with a much smaller boy. When he applied the brakes too hard going down a hill on the unfamiliar bike he flew over the handlebars backward and landed awkwardly on his head, neck, and back.

After assessing Philip's condition, Paul decided he had no choice but to have him airlifted by helicopter to a large, well-equipped hospital. The medical evaluation revealed very bad news: compounding fractures of three vertebrae (T 6, 7, and 8) and a piece of Philip's skull was broken off. Philip underwent extensive back surgery that day.

Once Paul transitioned out of his first-responder mentality, he realized there was plenty to worry about. But as a devout man of faith, he quickly found comfort in his religious beliefs and the generous emotional, practical, and financial support that poured in from fellow church members. Because his wife and other sons share his commitment to faith and family, they held family meetings, prayed together, and collectively supported each other as they navigated this family challenge. Talking about his wife specifically, Paul says, "We really knew we had to take care of each other, and I think it's done a lot to bring us closer." He also adds that the accident has led him to appreciate his wife even more.

Unlike some physical conditions and diseases that are marked by gradual symptoms and discomfort, Philip's type of injury required Philip, Paul, and the rest of the family to make a radical shift without warning. Suddenly, Paul was contemplating how to provide care for a child with a significant disability who had only hours earlier been a physically active teenager with no health issues whatsoever. Paul eventually would clean up after Philip as though he were a toddler not yet potty trained for what seemed like "eons."

Four or five days after the accident, Philip grew more alert as the morphine drip was lessened. It was then that Paul stepped forward with his reality check and a challenge for his son that ultimately framed their lasting response to Philip's paralysis. "I told 'em 'Look, you know, we can either be real depressed about this or we can have a good time with it. Which one do you want to do?' And he is pretty forthright. He said 'I'd rather have a good time with it,' so we decided that's what we would do. So, we started picking on all of the medical people in the hospital and really they loved it."

In the weeks and months ahead, Philip and Paul became a comedic team of sorts as they played hilarious pranks on unsuspecting medical staff. They also joined forces to create a clever and funny newsletter that documents different aspects of Philip's long rehabilitation, which they circulate electronically. Paul describes a few of their antics by saying, "We had taken a series of pictures with him sittin' in the chair and me with a four-pound hammer I was going to test his reflexes to see if he had any return out of them. And then, his next one I got a picture when his leg went into spasm and it came out like this. I was on the floor unconscious."

When Paul and Philip made their pact to embrace the situation, they entered into a new strategic partnership rooted in their shared faith and tight familial bond. A health tragedy fostered the need for their unique partnership, but its foundation was firmly in place long before. Paul had always had a loving, respectful relationship with Philip.

Four years after the accident, Philip remained paralyzed from the waist down, restricted to a wheelchair, but in good spirits.

Paul's extended account of how he and Philip have responded to Philip's injury is an inspiring tale that illustrates the reciprocal relations that frame the health matrix for fathers and their children. Much like Landen's dad did not allow him to feel sorry for himself after he lost his leg to cancer at thirteen—pushing him to try creative solutions to enrich his life as an active, one-legged teenager—Paul pressed Philip to adjust and stay fit despite his limited mobility. "I won't let him use an electric wheelchair . . . he and I agreed on that because we wanted him to be able to keep his upper body in shape. So, he does that. He's seventeen years old. He doesn't need to be going around on batteries." Paul also put his woodworking skills to good use by building a hydraulic powered "stander" that enables Philip to hold himself upright for short periods of time. As Paul says, compared to his wife he was "tougher on pushing him [Philip]" to have to learn to do things himself. They talked it through, sometimes arguing, but ultimately his wife deferred to Paul's "tough love" strategy.

Despite Paul's commendable efforts, Philip has probably done more to make the partnership a productive one. By showing remarkable courage in the face of personal tragedy, this teenage boy's ability to adapt to his new lifestyle has made it easier for Paul and his wife to manage their emotions and their demanding responsibilities. With a chuckle, Paul observes, "But you know honestly it really doesn't bother him. He's perfectly fine with it. So, with that in mind it's easier for me when I do get, you know, those kind of sad feelings to get past them." Although it's hard to fathom that Philip isn't bothered by his paralysis, one gets the impression that, at least in Paul's eyes, his son has adjusted well beyond what most people might expect.

Paul's story is one of many I heard about children being resilient and struggling to make the most of their unfortunate circumstances. Like Paul, many fathers spoke proudly of how well their children persevered despite facing significant challenges to their health and well-being. But many children are not as adept in adjusting to their atypical circumstances.

As I listened to Paul and others tell their stories about their children with special needs I found myself daydreaming about various types of "what if" scenarios involving Phoenix. Nearly a year after I met Paul and heard about his son's accident I was five minutes into a Sunday afternoon bike ride with Phoenix and his friend on a series of isolated paved streets that were part of a new development plan. Cars were not permitted on the roads so I let Phoenix pedal ahead a bit until I saw him bolting with his head down. My screams "Look up, Phoenix!" raised his head but were not in time to stop the contact. An image flashed before me of what was about to happen, but I was helpless. Phoenix barreled head-on into the curb and his fifty-seven pounds of flesh and bones as well as the bike went flying. He somersaulted over the top of the handlebars landing with a thud in a grassy, weeded area; his bike smashed onto the curb and street. The impact knocked off his helmet. Immediately, traumatic cries shrieked through the empty land as I rushed to his side. Fortunately, Phoenix rolled over and sat up as I reached for him. Sorting through the screams and tears I saw that he was fixated on his right forearm. 'Was it broken?' I asked myself silently. On sight and touch nothing appeared out of the ordinary.

The traumatic crying eventually faded to whimpering, and after a brief walk up the street to calm ourselves a bit we rode another mile. Within minutes Phoenix made it clear that he had had enough of biking for the day so we turned toward home to get an icepack and pool time. The pool lifted his spirits for the evening but his complaints resurfaced the next morning. Our early morning trip for x-rays showed that his bones were intact. Phoenix and I both marveled as we studied the bones beneath the flesh on his hands and arms. The doctor cleared him to resume his normal activities.

At my request, she reinforced the message I had shared many, many times with Phoenix: it is not safe to ride his bike with his head down. I had told him countless times that an accident like the one he had was going to happen if he didn't heed my warnings. Would this event do what my verbal pleas for safety could not? A bit, perhaps, but when Phoenix wanted to fly on his mountain bike in the ensuing months he continued to pedal from time to time with his head down. Post-crash, I could at least more easily get his short-term attention by reminding him of his crash. Now, several years removed from the accident, I still have to remind him to keep his eyes up when he's riding—even faster—on his road bike.

As we left the emergency room Phoenix looked up at me. "You know why my arm wasn't broken, Daddy?" I smiled as I correctly anticipated his answer. "Because I've been drinking my milk."

FATHERING CHILDREN WITH DEVELOPMENTAL DISABILITIES

Like Paul, many of the fathers I interviewed, and countless more across the United States, have children living with significant health-related conditions that adversely affect their lives. In the academic and social service communities, terms like *disabilities, developmental disabilities (DD), learning disabilities (LD), chronic illnesses and conditions, life-threatening illnesses, sensory impairments,* and *special needs* are common labels to categorize the challenges facing many kids, parents, and families.

The 1990 Americans with Disabilities Act (ADA), as amended in 2009, defines disability as "a physical or mental impairment that substantially limits one or more major life activities" for an individual.[1] ADA defines these activities to include at least the following: "caring for oneself, performing manual tasks, seeing, hearing, eating, sleeping, walking, standing, lifting, bending, speaking, breathing, learning, reading, concentrating, communicating, and working." In addition, these extensive activities include the "operation of a major bodily function, including but not limited to, functions of the immune system, normal cell growth, digestive, bowel, bladder, neurological, brain, respiratory, circulatory, endocrine, and reproductive functions." Impairments are expected to have an actual or expected duration of at least six months. Lastly, a disability is perceived to exist even when "mitigating measures" like medications, prosthetics, and other devices enable a person to experience the previously restricted major life activity. Thus, even though Campbell's insulin-dependent, diabetic son works out and functions fairly well because he carefully monitors his meds, he is still classified as having a disability according to the definition.

Disabilities come in many forms. Some curtail a child's opportunity to think and emote like his peers, others steal a child's ability to use limbs and organs as they were meant to work, and others snatch a child's hope of living a long life or accomplishing certain goals. Sadly, some disabilities are so debilitating that they severely diminish a child's emotional, physical, and intellectual capacities. Many parents whose children are not touched by some type of disability probably underestimate the number of families who are affected. Roughly one out of every six children in the United States age three to seventeen live with one or more developmental disabilities.[2] That's ten million kids, more than the entire population of New York City, the most populous city in the nation. Unfortunately, the number of children with a developmental disability has increased significantly in recent years, largely due to the sharp increases in the diagnoses of autism and ADHD. As reported by parents of children age three to seventeen in a national survey, there was a 72 percent increase in the diagnoses for autism between 2007 and 2011/12.[3] ADHD diagnoses by health care providers increased by 42 percent from 2003 to 2011.[4] As a result, more and more fathers find themselves needing to learn how to care for children who require special attention. Fathers are also more likely to interact with sons in these situations because males are twice as likely as females to experience a developmental disorder, and the gender discrepancy is most noticeable for ADHD, autism, learning disabilities, and stuttering/stammering. Efforts to help kids manage ADHD in their younger years may become even more critical to those who pay attention to the results of a thirty-three-year longitudinal study of white males published in the flagship journal of the American Academy of Pediatrics. The study found that those with ADHD as young boys had elevated rates of BMI and obesity as adults compared to their counterparts without ADHD.[5]

Until recently, though, little research and few social programs and support groups focused specifically on fathers with children with disabilities.[6] For this book, I cast a wide net to recruit fathers whose children experience various cognitive, emotional, and physical impairments.

Some of the more prominent ways a father is involved with his child include his initial assessments that something is not quite right with his child's health and functioning; his contribution to any health-related care provided to his child away from home or at home, including his efforts to advocate on his child's behalf; his approach to managing his own and others' emotions connected to the child's health; and his contributions to administrative and financial management issues surrounding a child's medical care.

The fathers' stories reminded me of what scholars say about disability—it is a combination of both the physical aspects of bodies that are not "medically normal" and the social forces that shape how people perceive, experience, and respond to these differences.[7] The government, health care industry, media, and other institutions as well as individuals in their everyday lives affect how people orient themselves to their own and others' disabilities. While the meanings people and institutions attach to disability specifically matter a great deal, there is also the matter of how fathers, as men, are expected to treat their child and other family members. In a social world where nurturance and caregiving are still more likely to be associated with women and feminine attributes, men continue to face various obstacles as male parents for typical children as well as children with disabilities.

Children as well as adults who have a disability must navigate a social landscape that has become increasingly tolerant and at times accepting of persons with disabilities, but, unfortunately, prejudice and discrimination still exist throughout our society. Identifying, understanding, and challenging whatever divisive practices remain helps define the field of disabilities studies.[8] We especially need to know more about how disability issues affect fathers and children as they jointly navigate the health matrix.

DISCOVERING A PROBLEM

In October 2003, Russell was a happy, engaged father to his two-year-old son Kaden, a healthy and active toddler who loved climbing and going down the slide at the neighborhood playground. By Russell's account, his "sort of light-switch day" as a father came on a "gloomy" November afternoon when he took Kaden to the playground.

[Kaden] was just in this really dense mental fog, he wouldn't climb, he wouldn't play, he wouldn't move, much. And I helped him up the stairs to the platform where the slide was and he just sort of, just was there in a fog, and I was talking to him but [he] wasn't really very responsive and he eventually, the platform . . . was about four of five feet off the ground and with nothing, it was just a step off into space, and I was standing there, but he wasn't really indicating that he was aware of me or anything and at one point, he just stepped off, into space, with no kind of regard for the fact that he was about to fall or anything like that and I was right there and I caught him, but, something was just, different.

Russell's disconcerting experience at the playground was especially telling because only a few months earlier while he was shopping with Kaden, Russell met a mother who commented at length about Kaden. "He's so aware, you can see it in his eyes! Mine just sits there. . . . He's tuned in, he's seeing things and he's understanding them." Eventually being told that his child had autism, and now having lived with his child as of 2012 for roughly eight additional years, Russell clearly recognizes that Kaden is in fact not tuned in to the world around him like most kids. Russell's experience with Kaden also made him more discerning when he had a second son who exhibited autistic symptoms. With his heightened sensitivity he was better prepared to grasp his younger son's autistic condition.

Certain features of Russell's experience with Kaden are familiar to other fathers who recognize key circumstances that lead them to wonder if there is something "different" about their child. For some conditions like autism and ADHD, fathers as well as mothers drift into assuming that their child is free from significant difficulties while they are infants. The symptoms for these conditions, as well as many others, often reveal themselves as children age and are perceived to be lagging behind other children developmentally, experiencing difficulties in performing basic tasks, or exhibiting behavioral problems.

Jake's first moment of concern that something might be different came when he was showing his seven-year-old son, Evan, how to shoot a basketball. As he pulled Evan's arm in to adjust his shooting motion, Evan's arm would shake and he couldn't stop it. On the spot Jake was able to confirm with his father, a doctor who happened to be visiting at the time, that something was not right. The episode set in motion several months of trips to prominent hospitals around the country in search of an elusive diagnosis. After receiving an assessment that later proved to be incorrect, the accurate diagnosis was presented as generalized dystonia—an often hereditary neurological movement disorder that forces individuals to have severe muscle contractions and abnormal postures. There's currently no known cure for it, but progress has been made on the treatment front.

A few years after coming to terms with Evan's disability, Jake was more knowledgeable about dystonia and on the lookout for signs that his younger daughter, Jessie, might also exhibit symptoms consistent with the disease profile. Ironically, Jake's signature moment with Jessie also came when she was seven years old. They were out for a stroll and she was walking backward and skipping a lot. After Jake asked her to explain her behavior, she reluctantly admitted that she was having trouble walking forward without tripping. Jake knew this was an unusual yet possible symptom of dystonia, so he and his wife took Jessie to get a formal diagnosis very soon after the episode. They now have two children with this disease.

When we talked, Jake was immersed in yet another round of surveillance for his third and youngest child who recently entered the age range when kids typically present signs of dystonia. On several occasions Jake has witnessed troubling things. He has even personally done body motion tests that have led him to believe that signs of the disease are present. However, when he has taken his son to be examined by the specialists, he's been told that all looks normal. For now, Jake remains vigilant but worried about the looming family health legacy that has defined his life as a family man for the past eight years.

As I listened to Jake tell his story I couldn't help but think that he has had an unpredictable, emotional journey as a father. The first diagnosis for his eldest son put dystonia on the map for Jake. Ever since, he has devoted himself to learning as much as possible about the disease while mobilizing financial and human resources to find a cure or at least viable treatment options. Although he seems to have adjusted well to his unusual experience, Jake has lived under a cloud of uncertainty wondering if his youngest two children would follow the same path as their older siblings. For some fathers, then, discovering that their child has a disability may not be a singular event. Over time, fathers may learn that their child has developed new but related conditions and some, like Jake, may even experience a similar process of discovering a disability with other children.

When fathers learn that their child has cancer, MS, MD, or numerous other diseases and conditions, a large proportion have typically already bonded with the child they had believed to be healthy. For fourteen years Paul developed a relationship with his son Philip before Philip was paralyzed by his mountain bike accident. Those years of building their relationship enabled the pair to transition more easily into a partnership that requires more time, effort, and patience from both of them. Even Jake had seven years with each of his two older children, seven years that helped him establish a connection with them and build their mutual trust. That trust has proved essential, because it enables Jake to incorporate his kids as partners into their treatment.

Although clearly different in some respects, Russell's and Jake's stories convey one of several broad scenarios involving how fathers become aware of their child's difficulties. They depict how a father might gradually begin to wonder about his child's condition even though, retrospectively, he can pinpoint a critical moment that led him to think seriously about his child's health problem.

Sometimes, though, the bad news comes more clearly, more directly, perhaps even before the child is born and before a father has even had a chance to bond face-to-face with his infant, toddler, young child, or adolescent.

One of the sadder yet inspiring stories I heard was offered by Nolan, a forty-six-year-old minister who knew long before his son was born that his child was going to have serious special needs. The news was broken to him and his wife before they had their first wedding anniversary. They learned at one of the first ultrasounds that the child would have grave abnormalities involving the heart, kidneys, intestines, and probably more. But the couple never wavered in their conviction to have the child even though a few doctors hinted at the possibility of terminating the pregnancy. Nolan recalls distinctly one young resident who expressed what Nolan thought to be an unusual perspective from a medical person that "this is the child you were meant to have—this is who he is." Ultimately, the baby was born deaf, essentially blind, not able to walk, subject to having seizures, and he required a feeding tube. The child was largely nonresponsive and could not sign. While the child required extensive care, Nolan and his wife had braced themselves as best they could for the eventuality because they had had a number of months to prepare.

In contrast, Steve and his wife had no warning of their child's congenital special needs prior to his birth nineteen years ago. The pediatrician told Steve within a half an hour of the birth "your son has a number of the signs of Down syndrome." The immediate details of the emotional upheaval are a bit blurry for Steve both because of the passage of time and because the experience, understandably, rattled him, yet he has retained deep impressions of having his world turned upside down. In a reflective, deliberative voice he describes how he felt immediately after his son's birth.

> Everything that was exciting and joyous and kind of a blur up till then, you know, it was like the bottom dropped out of all that and it became a totally different experience, just a totally shifted reality . . . it shifted to a nightmare I guess is what I'd say . . . when I learned that Brandon had Down syndrome and I was the one that told my wife, that was just one of those moments where all of a sudden you realize that everything in your life from that point forward is going to be different, sort of in the same way that I imagine when someone has the experience of losing a child.

Nolan and Steve share stories that illustrate how early, difficult moments can set in motion a father's caregiving trajectory. Unlike the majority of dads, fathers of children with special needs that are apparent prenatally or at birth are without those uncomplicated, cherished first moments of exhilaration—those magical times when months of preparing for the child to arrive are celebrated with an emotional big bang and the hands-on bonding begins. In these situations the practical realities of how disability is socially constructed in our society become real. Parents see firsthand how raising a child is going to be different and challenging.

BEING INVOLVED AND BECOMING AN ADVOCATE

The recent surge in the number of nurturing dads is vital to typical children as well as those with special needs. Nurturance involves being mindful and responsive in a caring way to a child's developmental needs.[9]

Fathers of children with disabilities can affect their children's health and fitness in various ways. Directly, these fathers can engage in exercise and physical therapy, give medications and attend to medical equipment, follow up with treatment plans at medical facilities and at home, go with children to health care appointments, discuss treatment options and protocols, and much more. Indirectly, they can advocate for their child to the professionals who monitor their health, fitness, and well-being; sign kids up for workshops, camps, and support groups; seek out information through friends, contacts, and the Internet to better inform their decisions about their child's medical care; and have thoughtful discussions with a coparent about a child's health care needs.

Regardless of whether a child has a disability or not, a father can try to develop a father-child partnership to improve the child's health and fitness. In some ways, though, the stakes of that partnership are highest when a child has an acute or chronic disability that leaves him or her feeling vulnerable. Aside from possible cognitive, emotional, or physical impairments, the child may face difficulties participating in specific recreational or school-based activities. When a father helps to identify and manage his child's disability it can lead him to build and navigate different types of partnerships with his child, coparent, and representatives in community agencies.

From the start, Jake sought to build a partnership with his son, Evan, by incorporating him into discussions regarding treatment options. The situation was rather bleak early on, Jake recalls, because the disease progressed so rapidly and aggressively. "He went from playing basketball with his arm shaking a little bit, to really twisted up and not being able to hold a cup, walk well . . . it was shortly after that that he couldn't walk. Not being able to talk, eating was difficult." Throughout those initial months of Evan's declining health, Jake and his wife carefully looked into alternative treatments. In 2005 they learned about an experimental surgery called deep brain stimulation (DBS) that had been approved in 2003 for treating dystonia. The procedure involves placing electrodes into the brain that are controlled by an implanted pulse generator (IPG), a type of battery-powered neurostimulator that is typically placed in the chest. The extension, an insulated wire, connects the electrode to the IPG and is positioned behind the ear down the side of the neck under the skin.

In Jake's eyes, because Evan was "really bright and kind of mature for his age," it made sense to talk to him directly about treatment options.

I remember just sitting down on his bed with him one time and saying, "What do you think about getting DBS? It could really help, you know, but they don't know anything and . . . you'd be the youngest person, in the country at least, to ever have this surgery. And it's basically you know brain surgery that you're awake for, for twelve hours." You know that's pretty scary for a seven-year-old. And he said "Yeah." He wanted to try it. . . . He was hoping I think that it would cure him, that it would help him so much that he could do everything. You know, play with his friends and whatever else. But we counseled him, you know told him that probably couldn't happen.

Evan improved noticeably with the DBS, so it appears they made the right decision. He was able to get out of his wheelchair, hold a glass and drink by himself, and do other things on his own that he couldn't before. Jake's hands-on experience with Evan also prepared him to navigate Jessie's circumstances in a collaborative way while reinforcing the partnership he had established with his son years before. "I learned to get her or him involved in every aspect of their care. That it's not a decision that their mother or myself can just make for them. We're in this together kind of thing. You know, any kind of decision, whether it's surgery or anything really."

While listening to Jack re-create his serious talk with Evan when his boy was just seven years old, I imagined myself sitting next to Phoenix on his bed trying to have a similar exchange. I wonder whether I could keep it together while looking at my child's transformed, "twisted up" body as we discussed the prospects of brain surgery. I suspect that many parents who have never traveled down this road have concerns like mine. But I assume, too, that most who have these talks find a way to give their child the confidence and courage to move forward.

An important challenge many parents who have a child with a disability face is to find the "proper" balance between pushing and protecting or pampering their child as they try to help the child adapt to the functional aspects of an impairment as well as its social stigma. The challenge gets especially taxing when the father and coparent perceive this balance differently.

Chad is one of many fathers who describe their intention to have their child become independent while not setting the child up for repeated failures, misery, or injury. Chad's first child was born six weeks premature and had various complications early on, landing her in the neonatal intensive care unit for more than a week. At home, she had a feeding tube for a number of months. But the big news came when she was six months old. Chad and his wife learned that their daughter was totally blind in one eye and had extremely limited vision in her other eye. By age two, the girl was diagnosed with a growth deficiency and has been receiving daily growth hormone injections ever since. As Chad describes how he deals specifically with his daughter's vision impairment he stresses how he wants her "to reach her maximum potential, and not be limited by that." As he talks about "walking the fine line" he ultimately acknowledges that "my tendency would be to push more than protect, simply because I don't want her to be constrained." Consistent with this logic, Chad has chosen not to alter his house and the furnishings in any way to accommodate his daughter's visual disability. He wants her to "interact with those variations in her own home." He believes this will help her be "better equipped for doing that outside of the home."

Beyond the home, a father of a child who has a disability can make a difference by communicating effectively with health care professionals who work with his child. These conversations can take many forms depending on the type of disability or health concern a child has as well as the circumstances associated with a particular setting and event. To be an effective advocate the father often, but not always, needs to establish an ongoing line of communication with the person or persons of interest responsible for the child's health care. If this is done well, the father can serve as a bridge between a child's treatment at home and at a health care facility. If it's done poorly, the father can jeopardize the quantity and quality of care his child receives.

Unfortunately, many of the pediatric health care professionals I spoke with agree that fathers are far less active than mothers in monitoring their child's health care whether the child has a disability or not. Not surprisingly, they also say fathers are typically less adept at providing a child's medical history and commenting on the child's symptoms. Both medical professionals and the fathers who attend consultations tend to lean on mothers to provide more detailed accounts of a child's medical history.

One very experienced pediatric pulmonologist, Arnie, notes that a significant percentage of fathers struggle with the daily life activities involved in caring for a child with cystic fibrosis. Such daily life tasks include administering antibiotics in one of several forms. In rare cases, bronchodilators and corticosteroids may be needed to reduce the swelling of the airways and facilitate breathing. Children who have diabetes as a result of their cystic fibrosis need to ingest insulin and manage their diet as well. These are just a few of the many challenges that parents who have children with cystic fibrosis encounter on a daily basis.[10]

Arnie characterizes fathers as the partner who often does not feel up for the day-to-day care of these children and estimates that mothers handle about 75 percent of the care for the kids. Nevertheless, Arnie and other physicians observe that many of the men who are less active in providing care and less visible at health care facilities are devoted, loving fathers. They spend much of their time working, caring for other children at home, and doing chores to keep the household afloat during chaotic times. Although many fathers spend less time with the child in the hospital than the mother, many health care professionals still perceive them to be good family men.

Despite this reporting pattern among professionals, many are able to recall a small subset of highly engaged fathers. Vern, a longtime pediatrician, reflects on his experience with mothers and the select group of fathers who are the primary caregivers for their seriously ill children. He remarks that fathers are much more likely to be "very detailed, very compulsive, very organized in terms of record keeping, in terms of understanding the chronology, wanted me to see their chronology of events, tracking doses of medications and so on." Vern refers to these fathers as "hyperactive," adding that they bring notebooks, computer programs, and spreadsheets to the consultations. For example, he recounted that when he was monitoring a little girl's immune system after she received a heart transplant in order to make sure that she did not reject the heart, her father would "sit down and he would bring in I mean years' worth of information. And I'd say we should try, and he'd go well you know back here, you know it was fantastic, it was before the electronic medical records. . . . He was gonna be sure everything was understood and that it was organized and clear and there were no screwups and that everybody understood the chronology of events and he knew what was going on too." Vern views these "hyperactive" fathers as being eager to be a copartner with him and his staff in managing a child's care, and he welcomed their involvement.

Vern's description resonated with me while I interviewed Nico, a forty-six-year-old stay-at-home dad. We talked late one evening via

Skype while he relaxed on top of his bed with his feet propped up. Eight years ago, he and his wife made the decision that he would consider quitting his demanding executive position in order to care full-time for their three-month-old daughter. Fortunately, the wife had a stable job and sufficient income working for a medical association. After a two-week experiment with the arrangement using family leave time, Nico found that being a homemaker was much less stressful for him than his job. He was keen on the idea of caring for his daughter, who had been born with various irregularities, including a condition in which her throat was not connected to her esophagus, which meant she could not swallow. These issues required surgery and numerous consultations for speech therapy, physical therapy, behavioral therapy, and occupational therapy over the years. Now, eight years later, he is still at home caring for his daughter and her five-year-old brother. From the start, Nico meticulously managed all aspects of his daughter's extensive care and is doing the same, though to a lesser extent, for his son. He has managed his children's care with an eye toward keeping his wife in the loop. "I would always take very copious notes, there were even times, even to this day, I bring a recorder to certain doctor visits and then she [wife] can listen to the entire meeting with the doctor going to and from work."

Campbell, introduced in an earlier chapter, has always taken an active interest in monitoring his diabetic son's health. He gave him his first insulin shot and has been the primary caregiver when it comes to managing his son's diabetes ever since. However, his involvement has come at an emotional price for him. This was particularly true when Campbell had to take his son to have blood drawn when the boy was younger.

It was very emotionally draining for me as well as for him. I mean, . . . there would be times when we'd have to come home and just go to bed . . . we'd just have to take the rest of the day off because it was that emotional for both of us. . . . there were times when I'd go there and it'd be me and another nurse holding him down and somebody else drawin' the blood and everybody in the room would be cryin' because it was so emotional . . . when you have your child begging you, begging you not to let somebody stick them with a needle it's . . . pretty deep. You know that's a big thing, so it was pretty devastating. But . . . it all goes back to you know showing the strength, the ability to show him that it's gonna be okay. . . . back then . . . I would, a month before it would happen I would just start having, you know, anxiety about sleepin' and everything it was pretty traumatic for all of us, it really was.

A child may be less likely to have a nurturing dad like Nico or Camp-bell if the child belongs to the unique subset of children with disabilities that one pediatrician, Bruce, refers to as having chronic complex conditions (CCC). These children are challenged by having multiple serious condi-tions that severely compromise their ability to function like a typical child. Nationally, the children who fall in the CCC group tend to be from lower-income families. Bruce asserts that "in those cases the fathers are very weak in the lives of those children." Responding to my question as to whether he and his team have developed any outreach programs for the dads of these children, Bruce confidently says, "For the CCCs, the fathers don't show up, they walk out [on the family]."

Arnie describes three styles of doctor-patient relationships presented in the medical literature that can be extended to the fathers of pediatric patients: collegial, contractual, and priestly.[11] The collegial frame of mind has parents working with physicians in a partnership of equals in order to monitor a child's health and apply treatment. Both parties respect each other because they each believe that they can contribute distinct and valu-able information to guide a treatment plan. In comparison, the contrac-tual arrangement emphasizes that the patient is a client and the doctor is a provider of stipulated medical services. Obligations and benefits exits for patients and doctors alike and each has some degree of autonomy. The priestly model identifies patients as expressing a kind of blind faith that doc-tors know what is best and will address their needs—the patient's auton-omy is secondary.

Arnie and other pediatricians I talked to favor the collegial approach for patients and parents alike. Generally speaking, he believes fathers tend to want the collegial style. I certainly got the impression that men like Nico want to monitor their children's care by establishing a partnership with the various medical professionals he encounters. In the Internet age, par-ents with computer access can empower themselves as never before with relevant information to have informed discussions with medical personnel. Yet, because Internet information can come from either authoritative non-profits (Mayo Clinic, NIH), mostly reliable sites (Web MD), or less reliable sources designed to sell products and miracle cures, some parents may have a distorted understanding of a medical condition when they interact with a health care provider.

All relationships between doctors and patients—including their parents—occur in a specific context and sometimes across settings. When we contemplate fathers' experiences as advocates for their children we must appreciate the reality that fathers come into contact with medical professionals in varied types of settings, such as regular visits to a general pediatrician's office, low-income clinics, ER, long-term regular or mental hospital stay, and consultation with a specialist in a particular subfield.

Thomas offers an opinion of what it's like to be the general pediatrician for numerous and different types of families continuously for twenty years. "We are clearly partners in raising their kids. And that's what I love about general pediatrics." He goes on to say that the key feature to being a good partner for a father in this setting is that "a lot has to do with listening, I think that's at the heart of it, is really knowing that I have to listen to what he's struggling with, and to try to help him with that. I think that's what is fundamental to him feeling that I can be a partner, I gotta hear him first of all."

Both Vern and Arnie have worked at times as hospitalists—physicians who provide hospital-based medical care for a sick or injured patient who has been admitted to a hospital. Arnie believes fathers are less comfortable in this situation. He projects men as wanting to be the decision makers, so, they feel anxious and helpless when they are dealing with a hospitalist—someone with whom they typically have no personal history.

Arnie speaks about the art of medicine and how he sees it as his job to satisfy parents. Thus, he consciously tries to include the father in the briefing session. But as Arnie describes, this is not always easy, sometimes because fathers are working at the time of the session or are not actively involved in the family's life. He also sees fathers as feeling the pressure of being men. Presumably, they are concerned about whether they are doing a good job as advocates, doing all they can to place the child in the best situation possible. Because the father is typically not trained to make medical observations or decisions, he resigns himself to believe that he at least needs to do well in choosing the health care venue and the particular doctor.

Although Jay, a middle-class father of four, never had to worry about a child who had a disability or long-term chronic illness as such conditions are typically defined, he knows all too well how a parent can struggle communicating with doctors who are treating a very sick child. Pensive and animated, Jay recaptures the uncomfortable exchanges he had more than a decade ago with several ER doctors who were caring for his son Rex, who was twelve years old at the time. Let's pick up his reenactment as one physician tells him that a burst appendix is the source of his son's sharp abdominal pain. Jay quickly responds:

> "Oh, geez, okay, let's . . . get it removed." "Well, we don't do that." "Well, what do you mean you don't do that?" "Well, a child, now, we don't, take the appendix out 'cuz we found out that there's more chance of a problem or an issue than it would be to just let it, control the poison, and then let the appendix kind of like, shrivel up, and then we go in microscopically and remove it," and I was like, astonished! . . . "What? What are you talking about? I had never heard of such a thing!" . . . So then, I said, "I want to talk to another doctor." So I talked to another doctor . . . he kind of like was getting angry with me, because I'm arguing the fact that this isn't the way to go. I say, "Well, I don't understand. Have I been living under a rock? I've never heard of such a thing." He said, "In adults, it's different, but kids, this is what we've found, this is what we do." So finally, I got the surgeon. The surgeon came down, and she talked to me . . . I said, "Well, you know, I guess. I mean, what am I supposed to do? I gotta trust you people. I mean, I'm not a doctor."

Exasperated by his predicament, Jay is far from establishing any collegial partnerships with the physicians caring for his son. He tries to advocate effectively on his son's behalf during this crisis, but, ultimately, he knows he's at the mercy of the doctors' professional opinion. His son receives a CT scan to make sure there is no abscess and a PICC [peripherally inserted central catheter] line is placed in his arm. The next day, Jay and his wife are instructed to take their son home and are shown how to give him antibiotics with a syringe. Jay's raw reaction: "It was like, scary! You're like, you're gonna do this at home? This is crazy!"

Within days, and after Jay's wife convinces him that she will be fine taking care of their son while Jay attends an out-of-state wedding, his wife calls to tell him that Rex "took a turn for the worse." She's taking him to the emergency room. Jay frantically drives the 450 miles to the hospital and learns that Rex is actually having his appendix removed after all.

Days pass with Rex in the hospital, but he's not getting any better. Another CT scan reveals that an abscess needs to be drained. Coincidently,

Jay, an electrical engineer, is supposed to work that same day on the very equipment that is being used for his son's drainage procedure. When the drainage tube is inserted, things go from "bad to worse." The doctor mistakenly inserts a catheter too far and breaks through the intestine wall. The result: Rex bleeds internally for weeks, but no one realizes it.

In the following weeks, Jay's wife stays at the hospital every night while Jay works, takes care of their other three children and the house, and tries to visit Rex every evening. During this time Rex has "tubes down his throat" and is throwing up blood and passing it through his rectum. Then, at four in the morning, Jay receives a call from his crying wife telling him that Rex is being rushed into surgery. When Jay arrives at the hospital he has a chance to talk to the doctor but still struggles to make sense of it all. Jay tries to depict his state of mind to me, "when you hear people say, 'like a whirlwind,' like you're in a different dimension. You're hearing the doctor but you're just like, not understanding." Jay hears something about Rex bleeding internally, that a portion of his intestines will probably have to be removed, and that he might have to wear a bag until the intestines can heal. Whether or not he fully understands the description is unclear, but he clearly registers the news as devastating.

In the frantic moments prior to the surgery, Jay feels helpless. "We were literally running down the hallway, just the bed-people all around it, you're running and they're talking to you and you gotta sign papers, you know, anesthesia, and all this stuff and the elevator going down, it just, swept them right into the OR." As Jay and I sit in his kitchen, his vulnerable eyes reveal the fear and confusion that consumed him during his family's ordeal. "You just, like standing there, and we just went back up to his room, and, cried, I mean just, we just cried and cried and cried, you just, couldn't believe, that this was happening."

And all I could think about was, that first day, saying, "Why aren't you gonna just take his appendix out?" and the guy saying, "Well, 'cuz this is the way we do it now. We have less complications this way," and here I am, sitting in my son's room, he's in the OR, literally, almost dead . . . maybe feeling like, I should have told them, "No, I want them to operate," but, you know, I mean, you've got doctors telling you, what's best, like I said, I'm not a doctor so I didn't know.

Now, so many years after the events, and even though his son ultimately recovered from his ordeal, Jay still second-guesses himself about how well he advocated for his son. Did he do enough? Did he ask the right questions? Should he have asserted himself more even in an emergency room setting? Because of his "insider" status as someone who regularly works on the X-ray machines, CTs, MRs, and other equipment, he learned afterward from people in a lab as well as from a nurse that the doctor who botched the procedure "wasn't very good." He also heard sometime later that his son was screaming during the procedure, but again this information was shared with him only after his son had recovered. He wonders whether he should have asked more pointed questions to the staff about which doctor was the best or how the procedure went.

I empathized with Jay's struggles to find his advocacy voice because I had my own stressful experience when Phoenix was two and a half years old and had his tonsils and adenoids removed. When I finally received the doctor's postoperative check-in call after what was to be a routine surgery, my wife and I were told unexpectedly that Phoenix was being prepped to go to the pediatric ICU unit. He was struggling to breathe on his own so the staff had to reintubate him.

Forty dreadful minutes later my wife and I entered the ICU unit for the first time. As I turned the corner into his room a deep fear and disbelief overtook me. I was shocked and could barely recognize my son. This energetic boy lay motionless in the hospital bed. He appeared so vulnerable buried in seemingly endless tubes, wires, drip bags, and monitoring machines. He was sedated, his eyes closed. What type of trauma and fear had my little boy experienced while away from me for these past few hours? I felt, as Jay had felt, totally powerless to do anything to help him.

When Phoenix's eyes finally opened they were filled with tears, fear, and uncertainty. We were told that it was critical that he lie as still as possible so that he did not move the intubation tube and aggravate his airway, which would complicate and delay his recovery. It was impossible for me to cuddle him or to even listen to what was on his mind since his mouth was taped shut and he was drugged. I was left to read his scared eyes as they begged me to save him.

I tried my best to listen to the doctor's explanation of what had happened and what needed to happen, but I was partly in the dazed mental and emotional space that Jay alluded to, when processing information is not ideal. My biggest challenge as my son's advocate was to stay on top of the nursing staff and doctors in order to figure out a way to keep Phoenix sufficiently sedated so that he did not damage his airway, while keeping the infusion of drugs into his system to a minimum. This was frustrating at times because the hospital policy was to have the medications locked up in a separate wing of the hospital. Staff not only needed to track down elusive doctors to secure signatures for the drugs but also had to leave the area to retrieve the drugs. If Phoenix was not properly sedated he quickly became tense and intent on pulling at his intubation tube. Ultimately, Phoenix was released in several days and was his energetic self within a week. In the long run, I have the stressful memories while Phoenix, fortunately, is oblivious to what he went through.

MANAGING EMOTIONS

Social scientists who study parents of children with developmental disabilities suggest that fathers are more likely than mothers to adopt avoidance strategies and bury their emotions.[12] Some explain this pattern by saying that fathers are more likely to express a conventional style of masculinity that has them protecting others while remaining stoic.

In the big scheme of things, many fathers knowingly or unknowingly manage their feelings about what it means to be a father of a child with a disability. Depending on the specific circumstances surrounding a child's health condition, a father and his child are likely to face different types of challenges. In particular, the signature features of a disability are likely to influence a father's response. For instance, a child's physical disability may be seen differently than a cognitive impairment. The former can prevent certain bonding opportunities if a father and child are unable to start or to continue to bond through adventures that involve hiking, biking, traveling, or playing one-on-one basketball. But a significant physical disability may do nothing to prevent the father and his child from sharing stories, having a lively debate, watching media, or playing cards. If a child has diminished communication skills, on the other hand, this may change the type of intimacy a father and child can experience.

Intimacy can, however, flourish between a father and his child with a disability even under very difficult circumstances. Hunter, a fifty-eight-year-old father of three sons, first became a father when he was thirty-three. His oldest son was diagnosed after a few months with Angelman syndrome. This genetic condition is marked by severe intellectual impairment, speech difficulties, a balance disorder that produces jerky and unstable movements, and unusual "happy" behavior that includes frequent and spontaneous laughter and smiling. Hunter's two other sons have no disabilities and eventually became highly acclaimed athletes.

According to Hunter, he has always been much more accepting than the mother is of their first son's condition. She refused to go to parent support meetings, and he believes she felt uncomfortable with the child. Hunter had one "spiritual talk" with his now ex-wife in which he asserted that he didn't want God to fix their son and he felt it wasn't right for him to pray to God to do so either. She disagreed.

Hunter penned a poem to celebrate his feelings for his oldest son when his son was a young boy.

INSTEAD
Instead of walking with you, I will crawl with you.
Instead of talking with you, I will find ways to communicate with you.
Instead of isolating you, I will create adventures for you.
Instead of focusing on what you cannot do, I will focus on what you can do.
Instead of feeling sorry for you, I will respect you.

Ironically, Hunter's fondness for his son grew out of the intimacy they shared when Hunter began to spend more and more time alone with him during their trips to see medical specialists. His commitment to his child and his self-confidence as a father grew as he continued to take on more of the responsibilities of managing his son's health care. Hunter was determined to provide his son with lots of attention. He quickly became the primary caretaker and a stay-at-home-dad, a role he assumed for his other sons as well. His first son started to spend lots more time in the pool when he was about nine or ten, especially once Hunter connected him with a swim team. Ultimately, with the support of the swim coach, Hunter was able to teach his son to swim in a lane and participate in swim meets. At times

Hunter had to get creative, even luring his son with pudding to have him swim down the lanes.

Sometimes we hear of inspirational stories in which a father and a child with a disability forge a unique partnership as a way to defy the odds. For example, in early March of 2013, Justin Reimer and his fifteen-year-old son, Eli, after ten days and almost seventy miles, achieved their goal of reaching the south base camp at nearly 17,600 feet for the world's tallest mountain, Mount Everest in Nepal.[13] Eli, who lives in Oregon, became the first American teenager with Down syndrome to accomplish this difficult feat. His proud father told a reporter, "For anybody who has a child with a disability or who is impacted in some way . . . the disability is not a limitation."

In addition to the form of impairment, the timing of a child's impairment can influence a father's reaction. If the impairment is identified prenatally or relatively shortly after birth it may be perceived differently than one that emerges when a child has interacted as a "typical" child with a father throughout the childhood years and perhaps into the teen years. I spoke to fathers who received bad news about their children in different phases of their lives: fetus, newborn, toddler, elementary school, middle school, and teenager.

For Russell, the reality of his first son's autism diagnosis increasingly took hold of him over the years. As it did, he gradually reshaped his fathering visions and expectations. He sought to place things in perspective and manage his emotions about his fathering experience. The new reality was a "dream-crushing thing. You have all these pictures of things you can do with and things you can share with him and then, a lot of that just goes away, and, you still hold out hope that maybe someday, but, as the years go on, one by one, those, all those things, it's like, 'No, we probably aren't going to go, take a cross-country bike ride together,' that just doesn't seem to be in the cards. He's probably not going to go to college." As Russell speaks about his son's limitations he also implicitly reflects on his own values and the type of child he would like to have in his life. Russell makes it clear that his own atypical personal and family history, particularly his experiences with a brother who was not a typical child, color his approach to processing the reality that emerged for him and his son over the years.

There was kind of some, some soul searching about, "Okay, if I were all-powerful and I could do whatever I wanted here, if I could just throw the switch and make him average, would I want that? Would I want him to be just like an average kid?" And, I pretty strongly felt that I wouldn't want to do that . . . he wouldn't be my child then either. A lot of what he's going through is, seems to be a much more severe version of what I went through as a child. I wish that he could escape the hard parts of that, but I also really don't wanna see him, you know, grow up to be a, beer-drinking postman. I . . . want him to . . . find his own place. My family, through the generations has always been a little bit on the outside, a little bit unusual either more mechanically inclined or, the photographer with all the nerdy stuff with the tools or the cars or all this stuff. . . . I would feel even more alienated from him if he were suddenly just, the kid on the football team, you know, third string, lineman, reasonably popular but not too bright. . . . If you pegged him as average, I would be almost as disappointed as, I feel with all of the challenges that he's facing now. Certain, it seems to be a lot harder for him than it ever was for me or my brother, my brother was somewhat challenged. He was never diagnosed with autism but I think certainly today, he would be. . . . He had sort of the screaming fits, you know, crying, refusals, will not do what they [teachers] say to do, kind of things that my kids go through a lot.

As we saw with Campbell and now Russell, fathers with personal experiences managing their own or others' disabilities may be able to muster more empathy for their own children who differ from their mainstream peers. These men, to varying degree, have some sense of what it's like to have others see and respond to them as being different. Thus they can relate to their own children's concerns about being different and stigmatized.

Russell's reaction to his children with autism, as well as the reactions of other fathers who have children with disabilities, should not be seen as responses that occur in a vacuum. As I've emphasized elsewhere, how children manage their own emotions can play a major role in shaping how their caregivers perceive and respond to them. When kids like Philip and Evan demonstrate resiliency despite the challenges of paralysis and dystonia, they embolden their fathers' spirits and encourage these men to sustain the father-child partnerships they have nurtured. Just as fathers can be supportive of their kids, the kids can offer support in return—often unknowingly and unintentionally.

TAKING CARE OF BUSINESS

Although a child's disability or sudden serious illness can force parents to focus on the child's immediate medical needs, the mundane realities of life are stubborn; they don't go away. Someone still has to work for money, take care of a house, pay bills, deal with insurance claims, and care for other children. These obligations may be reprioritized and redefined, but someone needs to attend to them.

In crisis situations involving a child's health, dads are more likely than moms to perceive that their responsibility is to pick up the slack and keep the household functioning, especially when a child is hospitalized. As a society, that's part of our deep-seated, traditional understanding of what fathers do. They are expected to retain their breadwinning role while freeing up mom so she can be there for her sick child. In recent decades, women's more notable involvement in paid work and their more intense professional commitments may have altered these expectations somewhat, but they continue to persist. As the traditional breadwinner in his family at the time of his son Rex's hospitalization, Jay knew he had to continue to work and help out more around the house because his wife was devoted to being with their son in the hospital full-time.

Often this commitment to maintaining the house limits a father's opportunities to be more involved in his child's hospital care and clinic visits for treatment. The division of labor leaves the father potentially vulnerable—he may be misperceived by medical staff because of his apparent lack of involvement with his child when involvement is narrowly defined as caregiving. However, some pediatricians are clearly sensitive to the bigger picture and realize that many fathers are concerned about their children. Many fathers try to be the stoic anchor for the family and take care of the financial and many other family demands that go along with maintaining a household in a crisis situation. But pediatric professionals also note that a minority do far less than they should or could.

Adonis encouraged himself to be a stand-up family man when he learned there was a good chance that his infant daughter might need a delicate surgery a number of years down the road. His daughter was diagnosed about six months after birth with a ventricular septic defect (VSD)—a small hole in the heart. No one suggested immediate surgery, but some anticipated that surgery might be necessary when she was seven or eight. A lifetime resident of the Philippines when he became a father, Adonis was concerned from the outset that the quality of medical care available in his country would be inadequate if his daughter needed heart surgery. For seven years, he and his wife constantly monitored their daughter's heart and consulted with multiple doctors before Adonis made the final decision to migrate to the United States in search of a better financial future for his family. After he had secured a job and been in the country for three months, his wife and daughter joined him. Although Adonis's daughter was fortunate never to need heart surgery, Adonis believes his decision to come to America eventually helped his daughter. At age fourteen, she was diagnosed with cancer that required an elaborate surgical intervention which proved to be successful. Thinking back, Adonis is proud of what he's done as a breadwinning family man and health care advocate for his daughter. As he sees things, coming to the United States in search of better medical treatment and health care insurance for his family has been his most significant contribution to his children's lives.

6 ⌁ COPARENTING

As an eighteen-year-old college student, Tony met and started to date a young woman named Christine. Although he says they only dated casually and "went their separate ways," they made a pact to check in with each other when they were thirty-five. Tony explains that if they were without children at that point they would "get together and we would have a child and have a family."

During the time between their college days and their mid-thirties, they talked periodically and maintained a friendship. When their thirty-fifth birthdays rolled around it was Christine who broached the "baby" subject, and Tony was quick to recall their earlier pledge. Since neither had a child or a spouse, they decided to implement their college pact. Within the year they had a son, Abe, who is now eleven years old. The circumstances that led to Tony becoming a father have created a highly unorthodox coparenting arrangement.

Coparenting has a specific meaning among family scholars. Mark Feinberg, a professor of human development and psychology, describes it as the "ways that parents and/or parental figures relate to each other in the role of parent."[1] Elsewhere, I emphasize how coparenting for fathers occurs when they "navigate the shared and contested rights and responsibilities that go along with having another parental figure involved in raising a child."[2]

Feinberg's vision of coparenting includes four main components: the nature and level of support versus undermining in the coparental role; agreements and differences on child-rearing issues and values; division of parental labor that involves specific child-rearing tasks; and how family interactions are managed, including exposure of children to interparental conflict.[3] Thus, coparenting can be expressed in positive or negative ways and captures both the style and content of how parents respond to each other and incorporate the child into their parental interactions. Although this model is designed to focus on how parents relate to one another in all aspects of childrearing, I target fathers' coparenting experiences in reference to health, fitness, and well-being.

Tony's coparenting circumstances are especially unusual because Christine approached Tony when he was in a serious cohabiting gay relationship with Sidney, a man twelve years his senior. The couple had been together for more than a year when Sidney first learned that Tony and Christine were thinking about having a child through artificial insemination, yet, as Tony says, "I talked to him since I met him that I wanted to be a father. I made no secret about that."

Tony continues, "I did want to fill Sidney in on what I wanted to follow through with" but Sidney wanted to wait. He jokingly adds, "He could've put off having children for another fifty years." During the early period when Tony and Christine were discussing how the child would be raised, Tony notes that he did not press Sidney to get involved but he included Sidney "on what was being talked about and encourage[d] him to add, but he was—he felt [like] . . . he's on the sidelines a little bit because he's not the father and not the mother, obviously." One of the main agreements Tony and Christine made prior to conception was that they would divide their time half and half with the baby.

In a separate interview, Sidney offers a different rendition of the circumstances that shaped how Tony first conferred with him regarding the baby pledge and then made unilateral decisions. Ultimately framed as a story of deception, Sidney feels his partner and Christine intentionally went behind his back to have the child. Sidney begins by recapturing the sentiment he expressed to Tony when Tony approached him about his interest in having a child with a longtime female friend. "No, we're not ready yet and I'm not ready yet, we're just getting to know each other. I'm not interested." He continues, "And four months later we got a phone call [from Christine], two in the morning, that we were pregnant and I was shocked and a little bit irritated to say the least that all of a sudden I had to consider that I was no longer going to be the main person in the relationship so soon in the relationship. So that's how that started."

Despite his annoyance, Sidney continued his relationship with Tony during the pregnancy and was even present for some of the prenatal exams and the birth. He claims he wanted to establish stability for this child because in his mind the parents were very selfish and immature when they plotted to have a child behind his back.

In the early years, Abe stayed with Tony and Sidney one-third to one-half of the time. Sidney criticized how the mother lives her life and treats Abe, and he believes Abe learned dysfunctional behaviors from his mother. Abe was diagnosed at age three with oppositional behavior and ADHD—sensory overload—and has been taking medication for six or seven years. Sidney claims that when Abe was younger, and made the weekly residential switch from Christine's house to come to the house he shares with Tony, that he and Tony had to spend a few days working through the child's aggression and anger.

Even though he is not the biological father, Sidney seems to have been committed to Abe's well-being from the very beginning, evidenced by his willingness to visit Abe during the week so he could sustain some sense of continuity. For a number of years all three parental figures and Abe would meet for Sunday dinner at alternating homes; those dinners no longer occur, however. Tony and Christine are currently battling in court to establish paternal rights and negotiate child custody issues.

Tony's account of the mother's irresponsible behavior and the coparenting difficulties he has had with her coincide in many ways with Sidney's views. It bothers Tony considerably that the mother has a poor diet, is overweight, smokes, and doesn't exercise. Not surprisingly, both Tony and Sidney disapprove of how the mother manages Abe's diet. Tony wants his son to be aware of his ADHD and to take precautions not to throw his system off by eating chocolate or sugary drinks like soda. He sees how Abe loses his focus when he consumes such items and he mentions that his son "goes to Satan" with soda. Because Tony personally feels some of the same things that Abe does when he eats certain items, he believes there is a genetic component. Unfortunately, the mother ignores these realities by packing cookies and trail mix containing chocolate in Abe's lunch, and she lets him eat and drink other things Tony believes should be off-limits. He admits that this "ruffles my feathers."

According to Tony, it's difficult to talk to the mother because she becomes very defensive and is a product of her own troubled family background. She was adopted by her grandmother but is actually the daughter of her eldest "sister." Because there was a lot of deception in her household until she turned twelve, Tony believes Christine is dealing with repressed anger issues that make it difficult for her to engage in cooperative coparenting. Tony's approach has been to try to figure out a way to say what he would like to express without being too direct. For example, he comments or asks questions to the doctor while Christine is present as a way to get her to see things in a different light, such as feeding their son sugary foods. Tony also tries to convey that Abe has the emotional development of a nine-year-old because of his ADHD and that it's his parents who need to be responsible for him to some extent, rather than assigning too much responsibility to him.

Overall, Tony believes he can coparent more effectively with Sidney than with Christine because with the mother "there's so much hostility and aggression that it makes you not want to approach and deal" with her. Being on good terms clearly makes it easier for a father to develop and sustain a productive partnership with a coparent.

Tony's experience illustrates that relationships can ebb and flow over time, with parents being more adept at coparenting effectively during certain periods of their lives. Similarly, coparenting effectiveness varies depending on what issue is being addressed. According to Tony, he and Christine coparented rather well during stressful times when Abe was about four years old and they were trying to get him diagnosed and treated for his ADHD. Tony and Christine arranged, sat through, and sorted information from consultations with different pediatricians and other specialists. Eventually they agreed amicably on medication as a treatment option.

At times, Tony and Sidney have had their own differences in their parenting styles, which requires them to navigate their coparenting. For instance, Sidney refers to Tony as a "hoverer," but Tony sees himself as "caring." When Abe was younger, Tony's top priority was to make sure he was safe, so he displayed a type of proactive and protective fathering. Living next to the beach, he had plenty of opportunities to make sure he was always right next to Abe when he was walking in the shallow water. He also made a point of being right beside him when he was walking up stairs and checked on him several times a night while he was sleeping to make sure he was breathing. Because Tony was the biological father, Sidney deferred to Tony's style of protective fathering, but he made judgmental comments along the way. According to Tony, Sidney would say things like, "Just chill out, give him some space." To which Tony would reply, "'No! I'm not giving him some space! If he goes under, not only do I lose my son, but Christine's gonna kill me.'"

Much like some stepfamilies, Tony, Christine, and Sidney struggle to assert their parental rights and communicate their different expectations about raising Abe. Managing this complex family terrain and developing productive coparental partnerships is no easy matter.

Listening to Tony and Sidney provide different impressions of how they responded last year to their concerns about Abe playing football underscores their situation's complexity. When I first spoke to Sidney he remarked that Abe "did football last [year] but it was too dangerous. We decided that even though he wants to do that we don't want him getting hurt." He goes on to clarify that the mother was also involved in pulling Abe from football. "We all talked. I was really adamant. I saw this kid with a snapped neck, a ten-year-old, it was stupid." Several days later, when talking to Tony, I'm told that Abe's "mother did not want him to play football this last fall. One of his friends did get hit, got a concussion, third one in two years. Not good. So she held him out. He wanted to play and I said, 'You know what, I wouldn't mind your playing, but your mom doesn't want you to play and I respect that and maybe next year,' so he's gonna play this next year, this fall."

Given these two contrasting descriptions, I have no idea whether Abe is supposed to be playing football next season. I also wonder how much stock Tony puts into Sidney's views on this matter since he doesn't even mention what Sidney describes as his being "really adamant" about Abe not playing. Whereas Sidney stipulates that all three made the decision to pull Abe out of football, Tony indicates that it was Christine's decision.

Most coparental relationships are less complex than this one. Tony and Sidney's relationship is also atypical for how gay couples enter into and navigate their parenting experience. Gay fathers usually adopt children; a small percentage use a paid surrogate. Still, there are family members other than the biological parents and stepparents/romantic partners, such as a child's siblings, grandparents, aunts, and uncles who are part of the health matrix because they influence the extent to which coparenting evolves in a cooperative or contentious manner. These ancillary individuals can also shape specific decisions that matter for a child's health and fitness. Similar to Tony's experience, most coparental relationships also vary over time in how productively the parents communicate about their kids.

THE LARGER CONTEXT

Coparents react to each other as they deal with matters concerning their child's health, fitness, and well-being either by cooperating in harmony, compromising on principles or pragmatics, or being confrontational and dogmatic. Whatever they do is embedded in a larger social landscape that includes cultural norms, demographic patterns, economics, health care policies and practices, technologies, and more. This landscape not only shapes the everyday realities that families face in the early twenty-first century, it also affects how families are perceived.

Perhaps the most significant feature of the landscape is what has become the new normal for an increasing proportion of mothers—being invested in paid work outside the home. This shift has had a ripple effect because mothers are doing less domestic labor than their counterparts did in previous generations and fathers increasingly are taking on greater child care responsibilities. Fathers are also spending more time with their kids, although they are still less involved than mothers.[4] So too, a growing number of fathers are stepping up to assume responsibilities generally associated with being the primary caregiver.[5]

What does this mean for fathers' experiences with coparenting? Because many fathers have either needed or wanted to get more involved with their children some have become more sensitive to children's health-related needs and are more likely to respond to them. It appears that more and more fathers, including some I interviewed, are becoming the "go-to guy" at home when it comes to tending to their children's nicks, bumps, bruises, and illnesses or the children's pleas for certain types of meals, snacks, or drinks. Some are taking their kids to the doctors and some are even booking the appointments themselves. As they become more engaged and competent caregivers for their children, fathers are better positioned to exert a more informed and perhaps stronger voice in the child-rearing discussions they make as a coparent.

Yet, cultural stereotypes that depict mothers as primary caregivers and men as incompetent caregivers still find their way into public messages about how families should and do operate in America. It was just 2012 when Huggies was challenged by daddy bloggers for the commercial it aired showcasing a group of fathers with their babies and the following voice-over message, "To prove Huggies diapers and wipes can handle anything, we put them to the toughest test imaginable: Dads, alone with their babies, in one house, for five days."[6] Some felt this ad was degrading because it depicted fathers as inadequate caregivers. Chris Routly, a blogger and stay-at-home dad, started an online petition and secured 1,300 signatures before a representative from Huggies contacted him to see how the ad campaign could be changed to make it more appealing to fathers. The wording was subtly altered, "To prove Huggies diapers can handle anything, we asked real dads to put them to the test—with their own babies, at naptime, after a very full feeding." The latter message portrays fathers as more competent and capable of handling their child on their own.

More recently, on September 5, 2013, I was listening to sports talk radio while driving to pick up Phoenix from aftercare. A well-known ESPN announcer, Scott Van Pelt, was making light of how he and his mother were going to be in charge of caring for his infant daughter while his wife was out of town for the weekend. The running joke between Van Pelt and his sidekick Ryen Russillo was that Van Pelt was feeling insecure about his ability to care for his daughter effectively. He stressed that his wife has the mother thing going on and is naturally better suited to care for their daughter. Van Pelt apparently was content to be a mother's helper, unmotivated to frame his weekend spending extra time with his daughter as a special opportunity. To make matters worse, Russillo chimed in to advise Van Pelt that he should just go out, have some drinks, and leave the grandmother in charge. This type of stale masculine bantering perpetuates outdated and debilitating impressions that men are innately incapable of or unwilling to be attentive, nurturing dads. Worse yet, it signals that the antifeminist sentiments reinforced by the antics that define the social world many teenage and young men experience, what Michael Kimmel calls "guyland"—hanging out, partying, playing with tech toys and video games, and watching sports—have lasting consequences beyond adolescence and young adulthood.[7] Unfortunately, the residual impact of guyland may sometimes extend beyond the early adult years and affect older fathers who cling to aspects of guyland.

Thus, despite significant changes in gender beliefs in recent decades, stereotypical images continue to set the tone for numerous mothers to assume a gatekeeper role as they directly or indirectly limit fathers' involvement with their children.[8] Gatekeeping tactics, which can begin prenatally, restrict coparents' chances to coparent productively. They often lead to fathers feeling as though they are unable to provide top-notch care for their children or are out of bounds when they attempt to do so. Acting as gatekeepers, mothers, and sometimes grandparents, can alter the course of fathers' involvement with resident as well as nonresident children.

When Hunter became a father with his first son, he admits that he didn't feel any sense of intimacy with him in the early months. He felt that outside forces made it difficult for him to connect with his child. The mother apparently took over situations and criticized him for the way he did things, such as changing the diaper poorly and making it either too loose or too tight. He describes her as "hogging the baby." Hunter mentions how the mother was once stressed out early on and took the baby to go and stay with her mother for a week, leaving him at home alone. He felt marginalized by her actions and was frustrated that she did not turn to him for help. Her inability to understand his disappointment with her leaving exacerbated his distress. Ultimately, he became more intimate with his son because of his own unilateral efforts to care for him, not because the mother promoted cooperative coparenting. But just as mothers may discourage men from getting involved, first as prospective fathers and then later as dads, they can also respond to these men in ways that invite or demand that they become more active. Mothers can help open the gates for greater involvement for fathers and stepfathers alike.[9]

Even though restrictive maternal gatekeeping can still be found in some families, other social forces are probably as responsible or more so for fathers' limited caregiving.[10] Simply put, many fathers have themselves to blame for not being a better coparent when it comes to their children's health, fitness, and well-being.

In most instances men have the ability to assert themselves as active caregivers if they're truly motivated. Reflecting on his preference to be a nurturing dad, Terry comments, "I never want to be that dad that just goes to work and does this stuff and doesn't have that connection with their kids. 'Cause if that's the case, why'd you have them?" Speaking as a father who shares custody of his kids with his ex-wife, Terry mentions how his children see him differently than they do their mother. "I'm the one that they are okay with. And I know that if they were ever hurt or really scared or whatever, it'd be my arms they would want to be in, and I know that that would really hurt . . . their mom, but I know that's the case." Because Terry's kids are as "healthy as can be" and their mom "is in good shape and she promotes healthy living," Terry has little reason to discuss his kids' health with his ex-wife. But when they do discuss something, he says they are able to "talk about it pretty well and work it out."

Terry actually does more coparenting for his own kids with his current wife, although most of their talks focus on the kids' education because of her professional background in the field. He values her opinion a great deal, in part because he sees her as a "really, really super good lady with a good heart; she's just amazing." When a father feels connected to a coparent like this, he'll probably find it easier to coparent cooperatively and thus feel good about the process and results.

That's what marriage and coparenting are like for Oliver. A father of two boys—the younger is autistic—and two girls, with all four of the children seven years of age and younger, Oliver speaks glowingly about his relationship with his wife—the mother of all of his children. "My wife and I talk about things all the time and I can't remember the last time we had a pretty serious, you know, difference of opinion or something like that. Usually we're pretty calm [about] the stuff we discuss."

Both Giovanni and his wife, Nanette, a health-conscious, athletic nurse, have strong personalities. As a result, they occasionally pursue different paths initially when they're addressing a health issue for themselves or one of their kids, but their cooperative exchanges and respect for one another almost always guide them, eventually, to be on the same page. Twenty years ago, Giovanni and Nanette separately researched the pros and cons of using a nontraditional homeopathic approach to deal with their eldest child's ear infections. Despite being criticized by family and friends for adopting this model, they successfully partnered with each other and a progressive doctor who whole heartedly embraces this person-centered perspective. Ever since, the couple has been consulting with this doctor, and no one in the family has taken any mainstream, allopathic medicines. Implementing this approach has required them to be more attentive to their children's unique mental, emotional, and physical attributes in order to arrive at an effective "constitutional remedy" tailored to each child. Highly interactive and observational, the homeopathic model requires the parents to be patient, to get feedback from their children, and jointly process their observations about the children's complaints, experiences, and personality tendencies. Nanette logs these observations in separate notebooks for each child. Because Giovanni and Nanette have home-schooled all of their children, they have been able to monitor their children's development closely over the years and integrate the homeopathic approach more easily into their lives.

Coparenting Struggles

Lots of fathers are not as fortunate as Terry, Oliver, or Giovanni in having a coparent who shares fairly similar views about issues dealing with their children's health and fitness. Many of these other fathers live apart from their spouse, and many do not have any custody rights.

As family arrangements become more complex, many fathers who have an opportunity to coparent must do so while negotiating their standing in stepfamilies, adoptive families, and in settings where they only live with their child part of the time or not at all. A nonresident father may receive little information about his child from the resident parent. He may be unaware of his child having certain illness symptoms, injuries, doctor's appointments, medical tests, and vaccinations. He may also be in the dark about his child's dietary or exercise habits. Even the nonresident dad who is motivated to be involved may struggle to keep pace with what is going on in his child's life if the mother or guardian is unwilling to keep him informed or is slow to do so.

Cell phone and video conferencing technologies such as Skype have surely provided many nonresident fathers with a more direct means of staying in touch with their children, thereby lessening some of the need for cooperative coparenting—especially when it comes to adolescents. One father mentions that his teenage daughter who lives out of state regularly calls him when she's in the grocery store to get his advice on the nutritional value of certain food options.

As a nonresident gay father living in the United States, Zeke has felt rather helpless in recent years. He's found it impossible to overcome the negative effect of his ex-wife living in a European country. The unorthodox coparenting situation led to his daughter becoming a smoker. When he was a young man living in Europe many years ago, he hurriedly got married after discovering that he had gotten his foreign girlfriend pregnant. Throughout his time as a married man living in Europe, Zeke's strong antismoking message rang true for his daughter, even though she lived in a country where smoking was prevalent and she had a mother as well as extended kin who frequently smoked around her. "She was on daddy's side through that process but when daddy was no longer in the picture, she picked up momma's habits," is how Zeke frames the story. Zeke made it clear to his wife and children that he was annoyed with his wife's smoking, but she persisted. In hindsight, he suspects that had he been more physically present in his daughter's life in her later teen years he would have been able to divert her from becoming a smoker.

Some fathers, despite living apart from their ex-partner and not living with their children full-time, believe that they and their ex-partner do fairly well in keeping each other in the loop on most health matters involving their shared kids. Terrence, a forty-six-year-old African American father of an eight-year-old son, points out that he and his ex-wife

> go to all the doctor visits together if at all possible. We both call each other when there's something going on. "Hey, do you know any reason he should be puking today? Because he is. What did he eat for dinner last night that could have made him sick? What did he do after school the day you had him because today he has a, bump on his arm, or a rash, or he looks like he's been bitten by mosquitoes or whatever." So, there's a constant communication around that just to be aware. Just to know what's going on because if he wakes up at three in the morning . . . you have a crisis you need to know what's happened in the last twenty four hours. . . . we do try to . . . communicate our expectations around lifestyle in terms of just, being active, and participation in activities and sports, and swimming, and playing, just doing healthy outdoor type stuff.

In many respects Terrence describes what appears to be effective communication between parents living apart. He certainly portrays his relationship with his ex-wife as being sufficiently civil and thoughtful to handle health and fitness issues for their son.

However, living apart makes it more likely that some specific health issues will create concerns for coparents. Even Terrence worries that his ex-wife, who is not African American, is less "hypersensitive" than he is to the diabetes and hypertension concerns he has for his son. Because Terrence is intimately aware of his family's health history, he believes his son may be genetically predisposed to diabetes and high blood pressure. Terrence is big on helping his son make informed, responsible decisions about his health and he occasionally reminds his son that his grandfather died from diabetes complications. When he and his ex-wife were together, Terrence talked to her a lot about these types of health issues. But now such conversations are a thing of the past and he feels that he's not able to monitor his son's eating habits as well as he once did. Speaking about how he and his ex-wife differ in their approach to his son's eating habits, Terrence says, "I am more concerned with being aware of what he's putting in the engine." He adds, "I really truly don't know what happens there [ex-wife's house] sometimes and what doesn't." For his part, Terrence regularly reminds his son that there are "things out there that can make you sick and/or kill you."

Health Care Professionals

Pediatric health care professionals sometimes play a role in keeping nonresident fathers in their child's caregiving loop, although they admit that working with parents living apart is typically quite challenging. Some pediatricians, and especially specialists who work with children who have serious health conditions, mention that they sometimes try to talk by phone to nonresident fathers or working fathers who can't make appointments. Some also ask brief questions of mothers to determine the nature of a child's caregiving environment, further allowing them to assess risks and assets for children. Is a father even available to the pediatric patient? If so, what are the father's concerns?

These conversations may be particularly important when a child is undergoing treatment for a serious ailment or managing a condition like asthma while splitting time between two parental homes. Pediatricians should at least know what products are available in each house and whether parents are sharing information about what they are doing for their child. In addition, getting a clear sense of whether there are dietary differences in separate households is invaluable for those trying to stem the obesity trend. Typically, though, pediatricians don't do anything special to incorporate nonresident fathers into the social circle of adults who are positioned to support a child's healthy development.

Unfortunately, only a few pediatricians have given serious thought to how they might encourage nonresident or resident fathers to be more involved in their children's care. Similarly, pediatricians have done little to help fathers foster a collaborative style of coparenting that would benefit a child's health and fitness. Only three of the fifteen pediatric professionals I spoke with expressed any sustained and focused interest in reaching out to fathers, and I had targeted those three individuals during my recruiting because I knew about their commitment to dads.

For over a decade, one of those pediatricians, Craig Garfield, an associate professor of pediatrics at Northwestern University, has championed the need for pediatricians to pay more attention to fathers. His interest in fathers incorporates his appreciation for coparenting because he believes "so much of pediatrics is dealing with parents' issues and anxieties and concerns about their child." While describing his philosophy as a pediatrician, he says, "one of the things I love about pediatrics is being able to . . . form kind of a team between the health care team, the parenting team, and the child and make this triangle of care for the child. And if you're not including one of the key team members, that is to say, the dad, then you're missing key players and it can affect the outcome."

In 2004, William Coleman collaborated with Garfield to publish a timely clinical report sponsored by the American Academy of Pediatrics' Committee on Psychosocial Aspects of Child and Family Health. This report, which is in the process of being updated, highlights numerous ways pediatricians can do a better job of incorporating fathers into how they render pediatric care.[11] Among its findings, the team outlined ten recommendations for how pediatricians could "reinforce the father's support of the mother or partner." One of those recommendations suggests that pediatricians can serve as mediators when parents disagree on aspects of child rearing.

Practically speaking, pediatricians can most effectively support coparenting and act as mediators when both parents attend their child's appointments or are willing to set up a joint appointment as a parental couple. This may be most important when a child has a serious, chronic health condition. Thomas, a pediatrician with extensive experience, says he has lots of consultations where he arranges to meet with both parents who have younger kids with problematic behavior or sleeping problems. "We'd talk, and find some areas in which their conflict, or different strategies were undermining each other, and I think a simple discussion of those issues was very helpful, so that they became more aware that they were giving a very mixed message to the child."

However, practices that are limited to regular business hours reduce the chances of getting both parents, especially working dads (or some moms), to appointments. Initially, Garfield offers a pessimistic assessment of the impact of the clinical report: "[It] came out to a lot of fanfare and press and not much happened after that in terms of I think pediatricians' perceptions of fathers." But he goes on to note that a trend in pediatrics has been for more and more practices to extend their hours from 7 A.M. to 8 or 9 P.M. Monday through Sunday. Ironically, one prominent pediatrician I spoke with who has a distinct interest in getting fathers more involved continues to operate his practice using standard hours.

Pediatricians who seek to achieve the "triangle of care" and are attentive to coparenting issues are sometimes confronted with situations in which one parent asks them to do something and another parent is openly opposed to it. One married couple that consulted with Garfield included a mother who wanted her child to receive immunization shots and a father who adamantly objected. Garfield invited them to come to his office without their child, and he spent forty-five minutes listening to and commenting on each of their positions, trying to mediate their concerns while helping them reach an agreement. In the end, they could not resolve their differences and the mother brought her child in separately at a later date for the immunization shot without the father's approval. By law, pediatricians are expected to accommodate a parent's wishes if he or she has sole or joint legal custody irrespective of what another parent might want. Pediatricians, like other health care professionals who work with families, can only do so much to foster effective coparenting. Parents, ultimately, must figure out a way to find common ground as they manage their different opinions and parenting styles.

In addition to residency issues, money worries and inadequate health insurance—sometimes the absence of it entirely—can spark coparental tensions. Poverty can force parents into a frame of mind that they must be more frugal than they would like about managing their child's health care and fitness opportunities. The parents may differ about how quickly they should run to the doctor to have their child examined for particular symptoms of poor health or injuries. Disagreements might also arise about how much money should be spent on buying sports equipment, registering for organized sports, or sending kids to sports camps. For those wanting to enroll their kids in recreational sports, limited funds may be a real constraint. Registration fees plus equipment costs can quickly make it prohibitively expensive for some parents to sign their kids up for organized sports.

When money is not an issue, fathers are free to follow their preferences about engaging the medical community on behalf of their child and investing money in fitness-related resources. Similarly, affluent fathers are in a better position to manage their own health and set a good example for their children by eating healthier foods and spending money on gym fees and other fitness tools and accessories. Although having plenty of money does not guarantee that coparents will avoid disputes, the affluent are likely to have fewer things to worry about and debate concerning the cost of health care and fitness. ·

Parents with an educational and professional background in the biomedical or fitness worlds are likely to have the knowledge and interpersonal connections necessary to influence how they manage their coparental relationship. Today, more fathers than ever before are coparenting with mothers and stepmothers who make a living in the health care or fitness sectors.

According to the Bureau of Labor Statistics, the following figures for 2014 represent the percentages of women relative to men employed in a number of health-related occupations: dietitians and nutritionists (92), dental hygienists, (97), pharmacists (56), physical therapists (69), physician assistants (74), registered nurses (90), nurse practitioners (91), and a wide range of health care support occupations (87).[12] Although women make up roughly only 36 percent of physicians and surgeons, women are increasingly entering the medical profession as physicians. As of the 2013–14 academic year, slightly more than 47 percent of medical school graduates were women, a huge increase from the 36 percent in 1991–93 and 7 percent in 1965–66, respectively.[13] The rise of women in pediatrics has mirrored this larger trend. In 2010, 59.8 percent of pediatricians were women, whereas the figure stood at 39.8 percent in 1993.[14] About 70 percent of mental health counselors are women.[15] Finally, more than 63 percent of recreation and fitness workers are women.[16]

These employment patterns mean that fathers not only confront the lingering cultural message of women as caregivers but also are more likely to encounter female romantic partners who are well versed professionally in matters related to health and fitness. Because of this shifting distribution of professional knowledge between partners, kids might be even more likely than in earlier eras to look to their mothers for professional advice and guidance on health and fitness concerns.

Clearly, lots of social life forces can affect how fathers experience all aspects of coparenting—including dealing with children's health and fitness concerns. But for many fathers, the quality of their romantic relationship may be an overriding force that shapes their coparenting. When couples have a healthy relationship they typically are more at ease discussing their children's personal needs and habits. Thus, they are in a better position to cooperate and address their children's health needs. They will also be better prepared, if called upon, to handle the stress that invariably accompanies a child's health crisis.

A cancer diagnosis surely qualifies as a traumatic health event for just about everyone, especially for a young person. When Adonis learned that his teenage daughter had a malignant tumor it frightened him. Married at the time, he worked with his wife to determine whether they should pursue chemotherapy or a complicated surgery that could potentially disfigure their daughter's face. In the end, they opted for surgery, and afterward the surgeon assured them that it was successful on all accounts. Yet, Adonis remembers that after the procedure his daughter "looked pretty beat up. Her face was swollen, not that recognizable."

Reflecting on the time after the diagnosis but prior to the surgery, Adonis describes himself as acting in a traditionally masculine way toward his wife and daughter. "In the back of my mind I had a feeling that I should be the strong one both emotionally and physically. Just try to stay on top of all our health but more so strong emotionally for them because they were the panicking ones and I was the more stable one emotionally."

Unfortunately, all was not well on the home front for Adonis. As if the news of his daughter's cancer was not bad enough, Adonis experienced marital problems throughout the months leading up to the surgery as well as during his daughter's months of recovery. Those difficulties made his journey all the more taxing.

When I asked him about the extent to which he helped manage his wife's emotions after the surgery, Adonis was quick to reply, "She at that point had another confidant and that was the cause of our marital problems. So there were three parties at that point and what also eventually caused our breakup and divorce. So I was trying to give her all the emotional support I could give her but I guess she was telling me at that point that it was not enough for her and that she needed someone else to confide to so she was also getting support from another person."

With little support from his wife, family, or friends, Adonis was largely on his own despite making several modest efforts to reach out to others. Adonis's story reminds us that the coparenting experience for many is tightly woven into the larger fabric of a person's social life. For those coparenting couples who have gone their separate ways, the quality of coparenting might suffer because those who once called themselves a romantic couple have lost trust and respect for one another. Some previous partners, obviously, are more equipped to set aside their differences to do what is perceived to be in the best interest of a child, while others still harbor ill feelings and cannot coparent effectively.

Technology

Technology is at the heart of another shifting tide in recent decades relevant to childrearing and coparents' decision making. Fathers, especially those old enough to have experienced their childhoods in a different technological era, often lament how raising children in recent times has been made more challenging because computer/video technologies have made the indoor experience more inviting for many kids. As Xboxes, Wii stations, laptops, tablets, and smart phones have become more pervasive, parents are increasingly forced to make challenging decisions about purchasing, using, and monitoring these technologies.[17]

As we wind down our interview, Adonis invokes a passionate tone while outlining the pitfalls of our high tech world for kids. He uses his physically active childhood of thirty to thirty-five years ago as a point of comparison, then comments that younger people today have a "more sedentary lifestyle." After noting the prevalence of current technologies, Adonis concludes, "There weren't a lot of enjoyable things to do in the house as much as compared to nowadays so there was more of an incentive for us to go out and actually play with other people outdoors and . . . now it has to be more of a conscious decision of younger people rather than like something that they have to do. . . . They have to think, 'Okay, now, I need to be more active, I need to go out and do this.'"

The new tech era has ushered in a set of robust debates about what this technology represents for young people's emotional, physical, and social development. Some individuals, like Adonis as well as me, regret how it encourages youth to adopt a sedentary and sometimes nonsocial lifestyle that limits both their interest in discovering nature and in being involved in physical outdoor play. Technology is also blamed for the rise in childhood obesity rates. Despite these elevated rates, others emphasize how these technologies lend themselves to helping kids develop their creative, analytic, and multitasking skills. In our electronic age, the argument goes, children need to be prepared to manage these technologies in order to survive and thrive. Parents clearly assume that it is critical for their children to know how to use computers well if they are to succeed in school and secure good jobs.[18] Some of these technologies can even facilitate "mobile health" (mHealth) for youth by using text messaging and other mobile technologies to deliver health care information.[19]

What is clear is that more kids today are regularly using the Internet. Ninety percent of youth use the Internet, and young people have high daily rates of some form of screen time and phone use.[20] In one recent national study of twelve- to seventeen-year-olds, 78 percent of the teens had a cell phone and about 47 percent of these cell users had a smartphone that provides access to the Internet and apps.[21] These percentages will surely rise in the years ahead.

Because these technologies are related to parents' sensibilities about their children's physical fitness, the exploration of nature, exposure to violence, and opportunities to develop social skills, they also have implications for coparenting. If parents bring different perspectives to child rearing that speak to what children need or should have, the fathers in those relationships will be challenged to deal with these differences.

MAKING DECISIONS

Parents make all sorts of decisions that affect their children's health and fitness. Many of these decisions are shaped by a coparent's input. Some of the more important decisions include: breast-feeding, encouraging and discouraging certain dietary habits, supporting or discouraging physical activities or specific sports, choosing a pediatrician, determining whether medication should be used for certain conditions or illnesses, managing health and safety risks, signing off on or rejecting surgeries, and exploring options for mental health counseling.

In addition to these key areas, coparents also navigate how they orient themselves toward their young child's "minor" physical mishaps. Such events are the ones that often involve a young child bumping into a playmate or object, or stumbling over a toy or his own feet. These are not the horrific, gut-wrenching moments when a defenseless child accidentally flips backward off a high-flying swing and lands awkwardly on his head and neck. They tend to lack any notable traces of dripping blood, abrasions, bruising, or swelling.

As students of playground life know, guardians react to their child's physical misfortunes in one of several stock ways. I call these the "alarmist," "inspector," "diversionist," and "ignorer." In the minds of some, the alarmist overreacts by smothering a child, often making the situation worst. The child's frightened reaction is perceived to be more of a response to a parent's emotional reaction than the actual pain or shock from the mishap itself. The inspector takes a serious but quick look at the child to make sure there is no real damage, then pulls back if everything seems okay. Often, the child is asked to deal with the situation like a "big girl," or "big boy." A parent using the diversionist approach immediately tries to get the child to think about other matters and to "play on" by continuing with a new phase of the activity. Finally, a parent can simply pretend to ignore that anything just happened so as to afford the child the "space" to sooth himself or herself. This technique is more difficult to employ when other adults are present because the parent will feel pressured to avoid the stigma of being a "bad parent." A parent may feel compelled to at least acknowledge a child's pain before someone else steps in to soothe him or her.

Watching a parent use one of these strategies, or perhaps some combination, is telling. But the sideshow performance worth viewing is when coparents jostle to invoke their preferred approach. When Phoenix first began to explore physical activities and sports outside, I typically adopted the inspector or diversionist approach. Unfortunately, these were often negated by his mother's inclination to shower him immediately with hands-on concern and kisses.

Although I think I've avoided the worst of the old-school "suck it up" mentality, I've tried to build Phoenix's resiliency and self-sufficiency in managing his emotions. Because I've always assumed that he would spend lots of time playing competitive sports, I tried to encourage him to differentiate "real" pain from the incidental, minor discomfort that is common in physical play and team sports. My approach to have Phoenix "play on" was sometimes met with a critical eye and incredulous look by his mother.

I envied the couples who either naturally fell into a rhythm of like minds or hashed out a compromise backstage that enabled them to display a seemingly coordinated joint response to their child's mishaps. Part of our implicit negotiation resulted in Kendra avoiding most of the situations where I was coaching Phoenix as part of a team or simply playing sports with him at home.

A child's personality may matter just as much as the parent's personality in cuing parental responses to a child's physical discomforts. Here again, a child's reaction, good or bad, is an important piece of the larger health matrix that includes a father's involvement with his child. For as long as I can recall, Phoenix has been extra quick and dramatic in expressing his discomfort no matter how inconsequential that discomfort might be. As a result, he places added pressure on me, and his mother to a lesser extent, to figure out when bumps and falls are really matters of concern during physical play and competition.

I felt a kindred spirit, then, when Bailey, a stay-at-home dad with three kids, mentioned that his oldest son, who was about twelve, at the time complained that his lower leg hurt and that he couldn't walk without pain. Bailey admits that his first reaction was "you're full of boloney, you can walk." But after a few days of hearing his son complain, Bailey took him to the doctor who explained that the boy had "overstretched his Achilles tendon"—a condition that sometimes occurs when kids go through puberty. The doctor instructed the boy to take a couple months off from his jazz and tap dance classes and to avoid any other form of exercise. Bailey had been reluctant to respond more quickly to his son's initial complaints because, as he says, "Jeffrey is very, I don't know if you'd call it fragile, but he overreacts when, he has no pain tolerance whatsoever, so he could, it's funny when he's out in public he's fine, he could practically twist his ankle and you'd never know it, until he came home and you looked at him wrong then he'd be saying everything hurt." This set of circumstances highlights the reciprocal nature to the health matrix; when a father makes an injury or illness assessment he often takes into account his child's approach to injury, pain, and discomfort. He may also be compelled to factor in what he believes his coparent will think, say, or do.

As I discussed in chapter 2, breast-feeding offers an important site for coparenting. Fathers can play a pivotal role in supporting a mother's decision to breast-feed before and after a child is born. Although breast-feeding discussions initially occur prenatally, additional practical and philosophical exchanges occur once a child is born and the mother and father face the daily realities of feeding their baby.

Fathers have plenty of stories to illustrate aspects of coparenting as they and their child's mother manage the logistics of breastfeeding. Bailey sent a detailed note to me after our interview explaining how he and his wife approached breast-feeding. Prior to their first child's birth, Bailey and his wife, Samantha, talked at length about the health benefits and pragmatics of breast-feeding. They also knew up front that the progressive company Samantha worked for had a breast-feeding room and other accommodations to support breast-feeding. This exemplary father mentions up front how he and Samantha rearranged a chest freezer in their basement to prepare for their child's feedings. He then adds,

> I labeled and organized by date all of the breast milk bags Samantha would bring home. I would then bring up the oldest, heat it on the stove, and feed the kids. Since Samantha worked during the day, I would do all the nighttime feedings. She would feed the kids during the evening, and mornings, but any 2 A.M. feedings were my job. . . . Samantha would pump whenever she could. The pump had a car adapter, so at times she would pump while I drove to wherever we were going. . . . Her breast milk got very low in supply quickly after she went back to work. I did my best to encourage her to keep going, no matter how little she brought home. I was happy to be involved in the process. It was why I was staying home, and part of the job. It was also important for me to encourage her to keep going. She had some postpregnancy depression, so I did my best to be there for that as well as take care of the kids.

Bailey's self-assessment leads one to believe that he took his responsibilities as a father and coparent quite seriously. He clearly shows how breast-feeding can be a jointly managed experience that is enhanced when the mother and father are committed to the process and willing to coordinate their efforts.

Navigating Special Needs

Another set of philosophical and practical decisions is particularly relevant to parents raising a child with a disability, but they can be applied to other children as well. Earlier I described the dilemma Chad faces in raising his seven-year-old daughter, who is visually impaired, as he tries to find a balance between pushing and protecting, between challenging and coddling. Although fathers like Chad often battle with themselves to figure out what is in their child's best interest, numerous fathers also manage their desires alongside a coparent's preferences for how their child should be treated.

Kerry and his wife deal daily with their unusual circumstances of raising four adopted children, ages eleven, fourteen, sixteen, and eighteen, who each have special needs of varying severity. Their oldest child has epilepsy; the second child has severe dyslexia; the third child has significant ADHD as well as Asperger's conditions, which cause him to regularly exhibit antisocial, disruptive behavior, especially at school; and the youngest child has cerebral palsy and is unable to walk. She has very poor fine-motor skills, doesn't talk much or clearly, and recently has been having hallucinations and has gone up to four to five days at a time without sleeping. Although Kerry seems remarkably grounded and calm about the demanding circumstances he encounters as a father, he admits that he and his wife argue a lot about how to care for their daughter who has cerebral palsy, so that aspect of their coparenting is fraught with stress. He tends to want to do more for her and is willing to let her watch a lot of TV, whereas his wife wants her to play with her toys. With the son who has the behavioral problems, the pattern is reversed. Kerry wants to push him beyond where his wife is willing to go in order to make him more accountable for his behavior.

Fathers may face a unique set of coparenting challenges when a child with a disability has one or more siblings who are healthy. Disagreements can arise between coparents when they have concerns about how the other parent is treating the siblings of the children with special needs. Family life and parenting practices are often complicated because healthy siblings of children with chronic illnesses are much more likely to experience emotional and behavioral problems compared to healthy siblings of children without chronic illnesses.[22]

Prior to his divorce, Hunter experienced coparenting problems with his ex-wife, who felt their second son was being denied certain opportunities and was getting the short end of the stick because of the attention his older brother with a disability was receiving. As Hunter tells the story, she overcompensated and enabled the younger son to shirk responsibility for his actions and he began to misbehave. Hunter did not want to pamper the able-bodied son, and he expected him to do his chores in a responsible way. He was determined to teach this able-bodied son to be independent and responsible and he felt the mother was undermining that effort, in part because she felt sorry for her son having a brother with special needs.

Concerns can also surface when a father is perceived to be spending too much time with an able-bodied child at the expense of not paying enough attention to his child with a disability. This became a bit of an issue for Steve, who loves to bond with his younger son by going on hiking excursions around the world. Unfortunately, despite Steve's encouragement, his older son, who has Down syndrome, is uninterested in doing any sort of outdoor physical activity. Steve notes that his wife reminds him that he spends a disproportionate amount of time and energy on his younger son. Given Steve's natural inclination to be physically active, and his desire to share special outdoor times with his younger son, he is torn about how to manage his own desires and competing responsibilities to his sons.

Expressing Control

As is true with many household decisions, coparenting couples sometimes drift into an arrangement, or they explicitly negotiate, which person is going to take the lead on health and fitness issues. Having a medical or fitness training background can give a person more standing, but availability also plays a major role. Having professional expertise does not mean a person will automatically become the primary advocate or manager for the child's health and fitness needs. Still, that expertise may affect how specific decisions are executed. In Clifford's case, he believes he and his wife are on the same page or can get there easily about their children's health and fitness, in part, because he thinks she'll make smart decisions for the kids because of her background as a physical education teacher.

In general, the dads who have some sort of medical background as well as the pediatric professionals I interviewed who are parents seem more reluctant to take their child to see a doctor when the child is sick. They are more likely to take a wait-and-see attitude and allow the child's immune system to do its work. However, when Stanley was married years ago to a nurse, he felt she "wanted to rush out to the doctor right away when . . . one of the kids was sick. . . . She was overly worried about her kids. And sometimes irrational about, I think, what might be wrong with them." I sensed that the rift in their coparenting was particularly strong when Stanley and his ex-wife were dealing with a sick child. Stanley recollects with some annoyance in his voice how "she'd wait to the point where I said oh, I think it's OK. . . . [and] she would get angry at me and tell me that I don't know what I'm talking about or that I don't care."

When I ask fathers to comment on any significant differences they have experienced with their child's mother or other parental figure about caring for their child's health, the majority of them say that they are more or less on the same page. Yet, a small subset of men voice strong concerns, saying they experience a lot of stress trying to manage their children's health and fitness while being at odds with their coparent's beliefs and behavior.

Zeke came across as one of the more disgruntled fathers who talked to me. Not only did he battle his ex-wife over her smoking, which he thought was a poor example to set for their children, but he also has vivid memories of their very different views about the role of modern medicine in their children's lives. Mimicking his ex-wife's voice, "They don't need that dang vaccine, they don't need a flu shot, they don't need a pneumonia shot, they don't need that tetanus shot, why are you doing that, they don't need that." She apparently was concerned that these shots would make their kids sick. Zeke and his ex-wife even had a major confrontation about whether to circumcise their son. In the end, the boy was not circumcised and Zeke believes he lost the battle because it was "her hospital, her country."

Although the friction between parents over standard childhood vaccines did not surface in my interviews outside of Zeke's story, this emotionally charged issue, given added visibility in 2010 by the PBS *Frontline* documentary, "The Vaccine War," can potentially place some couples in a precarious spot.[23] Celebrities like Jim Carrey and Jenny McCarthy raised the visibility of the vaccine debate in recent years, arguing that vaccines can lead to autism. McCarthy believes there is a link between vaccines and autism, stating that vaccines were a precursor to her son's autism. Public debate about childhood vaccinations was reinvigorated in 2015 and 2016 when many presidential candidates, most notably republican candidate at the time Donald

Trump, challenged the standard schedule by which vaccines are delivered to young children. Some candidates suggested parents should have the right to refuse to have their children vaccinated.[24]

But not all couples have two partners who share the same view on this issue as Carrey and McCarthy did when they were partnered. And I suspect that many couples, prior to becoming pregnant with their first child, do not even discuss their personal opinions about the medical risks and benefits associated with having their very young child vaccinated. For a select sub-set, this oversight can produce an unexpected confrontation when a child is conceived or born. Tensions may also surface in unexpected ways when couples separate and become anxious about the spread of disease once they are "forced" to expose their children to what they perceive to be risky situ-ations, such as sending them to another household or receiving them into their own homes during child visitations.

Coparental rift can also emerge over the acceptance of vaccines designed for adolescents, for example, the HPV (human papillomavirus infection), Tdap (tetanus, diphtheria, and pertussis, popularly known as whooping cough), and MCV4 (bacterial meningitis). By far the most parental worry and displeasure has been reported in connection with school mandated vaccinations for HPV.[25] While it is unclear how often parents disagree about whether their child should receive the HPV vaccine, parents are probably more emotionally and morally invested in their position about this vaccine because it targets HPV-related diseases (genital warts and cervical cancer) that can be transmitted through sexual contact. Unlike in Zeke's case where both the dad and mom held strong beliefs about a course of action they wanted to pursue with their children, some couples negotiate a coparent-ing scenario with one person committed to a position and the other having either mixed or less tightly held views. I found myself in this latter situa-tion when Phoenix entered kindergarten and information about the annual FluMist shot was distributed to parents. The marketing line was "FluMist is safe, effective and free, and immunizing children helps protect the family and the entire community from the flu." I initially thought it was worthy of an open discussion with Kendra, but she was of a different mind. Armed with the expertise that comes with her Ph.D. in microbiology and cell sci-ence, she forcefully asserted that it would be irresponsible to subject Phoe-nix to the health risks associated with a live attenuated influenza vaccine that, in her opinion, is poorly developed and tested, despite FDA approval.

Feeling that I was out of my league in terms of the science of how the vaccine was created, I deferred to her judgment and hoped for the best. Then, and now, I recognize that I don't feel at ease with biochemistry and that I continue to marvel at my wife's ability to grasp seemingly complex, natural science principles. Thus our exchange illustrates that one aspect of coparenting involves the parents' approach to acknowledging their own and their partners' strengths and weaknesses in the course of managing their children's health, fitness, and well-being.

Sometimes those strengths and weaknesses are obvious, as Rafael's story shows. Rafael and his wife, who is visually impaired, have a thirteen-year-old daughter. From the early days of his child being in the ICU because of a heart murmur and difficulties breathing, Rafael has consciously tried to describe different aspects of the child's life and surroundings to his wife so that she could more fully embrace her experience as a mother. When their daughter started to crawl it became even more important for Rafael to narrate what the baby was doing and where she was. He learned to become very descriptive because his wife wanted lots of information. Rafael has played recreational sports with his daughter such as basketball, baseball, football, and lots of play in the yard. It's understood that he should take on more responsibility for these situations because his wife cannot participate as actively. He is also in charge of measuring and dispensing medications for his daughter.

When it comes to parents addressing ADHD and autism, Thomas—the pediatrician introduced earlier—estimates that roughly 50 to 60 percent of parents tend to agree on a treatment strategy from the very beginning. Another 30 percent are unsure what to do, but they try to work things out. His job becomes extremely difficult when dealing with the remaining 10 or 20 percent he estimates are at "loggerheads with one another." The latter pattern—parents being on opposite poles—is more common when children have ADHD.

Compared to a circumcision, immunization, or medication decision, deliberations about a kid's diet may seem trivial. However, negotiations about what a kid should consume or is allowed to eat and drink can be a daily adventure. Dietary decisions, then, may actually create more friction over the long haul than seemingly more critical matters like a circumcision or an immunization shot if a father and coparent disagree. For example, when coparents don't see eye to eye on the ethical or health virtues of encouraging a child to be a vegetarian, the rift can make coparenting quite challenging. Family mealtime rituals at home and in public can morph into anxiety-laced events as coparents brace for awkward, tense moments—with one parent ordering a sirloin steak or hamburger while the other parent and the child order vegetarian meals. The vegetarian parent may feel disrespected and uncomfortable knowing the child is caught in the middle.

So too differing perceptions about what constitutes "junk food" and how important it is for a child to avoid it can trigger friction. Coparents may feel pressure to come to a resolution about how their child should eat, but they may be unable to arrive at a permanent solution. Ironically, even though John is overweight and smokes he takes issue with his wife's buying junk food at the store. Because she tends to cave into the kids' requests when they accompany her, John makes a point of trying to go shopping with them whenever he can.

SETTING A COPARENTING EXAMPLE

Dads often talk about setting a good example when describing what they've done well or what they want to do better to improve their child's health and fitness. Many frame this sentiment as a personal goal, but it often has a coparenting angle as well. Common sense tells us that children will be swayed more if they see two parents rather than one or none making a commitment to taking care of their mind and body by eating well and exercising regularly.

The kids in Giovanni's physically active household have been exposed since birth to parents who value a healthy, athletic lifestyle. Giovanni and his wife have modeled this lifestyle through their exercise routines and eating habits. "I train and race, five, six days a week. So they see it all the time. Mama trains, many days a week, probably five days a week easily and . . . she's been top female finisher in a number of different races, obstacle, mostly obstacle racing and stuff like that. She's just a good runner, good athlete, good swimmer, good biker." Although Giovanni says that he and his wife have "never forced the kids to exercise," they placed all five of their kids into organized sports at very young ages. They've also spent countless hours coaching and training their kids in different sports.

One facet of coparenting for this couple, and others like them, is coordinating their personal, family, and work schedules in order to make sure they have the time to transport kids to practices and games, prepare nutritious meals, research athletic programs, register kids for different activities, and buy sporting gear. Some of what they do in a family context resembles parallel coparenting; they often exercise with or talk to their kids without the other parent present.

When both parents simultaneously engage their children in a health-related activity, this can be thought of as a form of collaborative coparenting. In this instance, a father and the coparent entertain a family fitness model by jointly discussing ideas with their kids about healthy living or exercising together. A couple might plan hiking excursions as part of family vacations, arrange bike rides and walks with the kids after dinner, or do video exercise workouts with them. However, with increasing numbers of dual-income couples pressed for time, and many kids with busy school and social calendars, parents are often challenged to find the time to exercise as a couple with their children.

It may matter little whether fathers are part of a couple that sets an example in a parallel or simultaneous fashion, or a bit of both. What is likely to matter more is whether children are exposed to a consistent, observable message that their parents are personally committed to a healthy style of living. Of course, hearing fathers or mothers "talk the talk" of healthy living is unlikely to be as powerful as watching parents "walk the walk" as they bike, run, swim, play tennis, do aerobics and yoga, hike, or participate in any number of other pro-health physical activities. Watching parents arrange and eat a healthy, well-balanced diet while minimizing or rejecting junk food can have a lasting impression as well. Ideally, fathers are going to be in the best position if they can collaborate with another parent to send a pro-health message to their kids. When children hear their parents supporting one another in their pro-health message it is likely to reinforce its appeal for some kids.

My personal experience and interviews tell me that kids can learn to adopt a healthy lifestyle in various family settings. My parents never exercised with me individually or as a couple, although as I've mentioned my dad invested some time in my younger years, allowing me to practice my football and baseball skills with him. I also never saw my parents exercise on their own or together. Yet my parents (mostly my mother) took the initiative to sign me up and take me to practices and games early in my life. They coparented well enough to make those early opportunities for formal sports available to me. It was that exposure to an athletically oriented peer culture, plus my shared time watching sports with my dad, that fostered my own inner drive to develop a lifelong commitment to exercise and fitness.

Like me, a number of the healthy, physically active fathers I interviewed overcame their experience with parents who were either overweight, sedentary, smokers, heavy drinkers, or fond of unhealthy diets. Relatively few kids have the luxury of having parents like Giovanni and Nanette who collaboratively impart healthy habits and inspire them to live a healthy life. Fortunately, a substantial number of young people have parents who are moderately active and encourage their children to eat reasonably healthy food.

Oftentimes, parents' ability to coparent successfully is intertwined with elements of the health matrix that extend beyond family borders. Fathers, working individually or as part of a coparenting team with doctors, nurses, private therapists, teachers, coaches, school counselors, fitness trainers, and other professionals in the community who monitor young people's health and fitness can enhance their children's lives.

7 ⇥ MAKING PROACTIVE DADS

ONE HOT AUGUST afternoon in 2013, Phoenix and I spent several hours riding mountain bikes to different playgrounds on the southwest side of town. I had learned a few weeks earlier that I could entice my six-year-old son to take long rides if we negotiated a mental map of playgrounds to visit in the vicinity. This Sunday we arrived at our last stop, Hamstead Park, with little time to spare before we needed to head home. Twenty minutes earlier Phoenix had experimented with a jumping dismount from a seated position off a low-flying swing at another playground. Because I felt he was not focused enough on making a safe landing I pulled a promise from him that he had to pay more attention if he wanted to "swing jump" at Hamstead. I also instructed him to keep his helmet on, partly because we were in a rush, partly because I knew he wanted to swing jump.

On his first jump he flailed his legs and arms around in midair like a monkey. That maneuver stirred my protective impulses, so I encouraged him to tone it down. "Just clap your hands once before you land," I told him.

He agreed and dismounted successfully the next time with a little clap right before executing a perfect landing. All was good, or so I thought.

After climbing back on the seat he went into his upward swing motion as he had done countless times. But this time something went terribly wrong and Phoenix accidentally flipped backward with his feet pointing upward. With his helmet in place, he did a face plant into the sand.

The next day, his pediatrician concluded that he probably had a "very slight concussion" and that it would be wise to restrict his exercise, sports activity, rough-and-tumble play, and video consumption until he was headache-free for five days. I complied and entered into an eleven-day stretch that culminated in his doctor and I concluding that Phoenix was fudging his answers to my questions about how his head felt so that he could spend more time indoors doing fantasy play. Because I felt good about the partnership I had forged with Phoenix's only general pediatrician since birth, I trusted her judgment and we lifted his physical restrictions. Two days later he did his first official kids' triathlon.

There's no way to know for sure if his wearing a helmet prevented a more serious injury, but I was glad I had asked Phoenix to keep it on. Despite Phoenix's mishap, I was content that I had been sufficiently proactive in balancing the risks of physical activity with the rewards that come with challenging the human body in play and sport. From years of observing parents on playgrounds I knew I was one of the most, if not the most, vigilant in monitoring my son's activities even though I tend to ask him to play on after his minor falls and bumps.

When I shared my experience with a graduate student and friend, Justin Hendricks, a cycling enthusiast and father of two young children, he sent me a detailed e-mail about the struggles bike safety advocates have had with getting safer helmets for kids as well as adults.[1] He educated me, telling me that Lazer was the only company at the time to make children's helmets with the MIPS system—one that is touted to help prevent or lessen the effects of low-impact crashes that are the typical causes of concussions. What Justin wrote next was provocative: "Personally, I think this is an especially interesting and important area that is suited to fathers and their involvement in advocating for children's health and safety. And it likely won't change unless cyclist dads, as well as dads concerned about head injuries, take some kind of action. I admit that I should probably look for some kind of group to get involved in as I think this is a particularly important intersection between my interests."

His words reminded me of how I have encouraged men—fathers especially—to be more attentive to ways they can make a difference for their children as well as other kids.[2] Compared to fathers, mothers have done a much better job formally and informally mobilizing themselves as child advocates. Mothers Against Drunk Driving (MADD), for instance, is one of the most respected nonprofits in America; it was founded in 1980 by Beckie Brown, a mother who lost her eighteen-year-old son from injuries suffered in a crash involving a drunk driver.[3] MADD has been instrumental in changing state and federal policies that affect alcohol, drugs, and traffic safety.[4] Although this organization has increasingly appealed to men as well as women, the leadership and volunteer base consisted largely of women in the early years and has been made up primarily of women ever since.

Could fathers actually mobilize to improve helmet safety for kids and adults? And to what extent will men and fathers continue to play a role in pushing for additional reforms in how head trauma injuries are treated in recreational and professional sports for kids and adults alike? Slowly but surely, men and fathers are transforming their macho views as the social movement to rethink risk taking in sports unfolds.

The subtle shift in how more men are thinking about head trauma and their physical safety in general can be witnessed across various sports and is affected by numerous circumstances. For example, Chris Errico, a former research assistant, races motocross and teaches youth to ride as well. His two young daughters and wife have insisted that when he rides he must wear a Leatt brace—a device designed to prevent spinal cord injury. Despite people's concerns that the brace limits mobility or that it supposedly hasn't been shown to save a person's neck, Chris has acquiesced to their wishes. He even encourages the kids he trains to wear one.

I wrote this book to challenge men, fathers in particular, to be more proactive in how they deal with health, fitness, and well-being issues for themselves and their children. Sometimes when men talk to other men about these topics they can open themselves up to new ideas, become more mindful of taking care of their bodies, and reinforce for themselves and others how dads can make a difference in their children's lives.[5] Men stand to gain by having more meaningful conversations about health, fitness, and child care with women and mothers as well.

Ideally, the men and fathers who talk to one another will share insights that ultimately improve their health and fitness and their children's well-being. The muddled reality, though, is that the information and advice men provide each other will be packaged in many forms and reflect competing perspectives. Contrasting messages can be shared about all sorts of matters, such as: Is tackle football safe? Does a particular medication work? Is it okay to expose children to guns? Is a specific diet or therapy helpful? Should children be vaccinated? Is it fine for children to lift weights and run long distances? In the big picture, because intelligent, reasonable people will debate what constitutes good advice, the quality and direction of any specific advice may be less important than increasing the number of conversations men have about these issues. What matters most is whether men and fathers develop a more proactive approach to health and fitness. Will they ask more questions and have more talks about these issues with their friends, family, and health care professionals?

Men can navigate the health matrix more effectively as fathers when they understand its scope, how they fit into it, and how they are affected by it. One aspect of men's understanding includes their self-awareness about their own health and fitness. Clearly, much can be done to improve the state of health among American men. Social initiatives are needed that get men to look inward and take specific steps to improve and sustain their personal well-being—for their sake as well as others' peace of mind.

Another avenue to improve men's understanding of the health matrix is to get them to appreciate more fully their actual and potential roles in the different types of health-oriented partnerships showcased throughout this book (father-child, coparents, a father and community organizations, and community organizations interacting with other such organizations). When fathers take a proactive approach to fathering they prepare themselves to be more effective partners with their children, coparents, and professionals working in community organizations devoted to children.

It's not just men and fathers who need to be challenged, though; we need to convince stakeholders who control our health organizations and other social institutions that it is in the public's best interest to incorporate men more fully into children's health matrices. We should celebrate men who personally transform their lives and become more attentive to their children's health and fitness, but we must not stop there. The prospects for a groundswell of men changing one by one are brighter if an ideological shift is reinforced by social supports that are woven seamlessly into the networks and activities that touch fathers' and children's lives.

PERSONALIZING GOOD HEALTH AND FITNESS

In earlier chapters, I highlighted how fathers often establish their perspectives and habits for health and fitness—good and bad—long before they have children. Logic tells us, then, that if we want dads to embrace healthy lifestyles and to promote the same for their children, we should get boys and young adult men to think more responsibly about their bodies and minds before they become fathers. If we expect individuals and couples to be self-sufficient financially before they have kids, should we not be willing to urge fathers and mothers alike to establish good health habits prior to becoming a parent? Surely adopting such healthy habits reflects a proactive, conscientious style of parenting. The stark reality is that when babies are born to parents who are sedentary, struggle with weight or mental health issues, eat poorly, smoke, abuse alcohol or drugs, or take extreme risks with their bodies, infants and children are more susceptible to bad health outcomes. So efforts to promote healthy behaviors for youth and young adults can have implications well beyond the immediate target group.

My sentiments are consistent with the message once championed by the The Boys Initiative which was founded in 2008 and was active for roughly seven years. This national coalition of researchers, community leaders, and others explicitly recognized that adult males are fundamentally influenced by their experiences as boys. Its mission was to "ensure that boys are prepared for rewarding and fulfilling lives that include economically valuable employment, successful relationships and marriage, responsible fatherhood, contribution to their communities and emotional health and happiness."[6] This nonprofit organization used various strategies to improve young males' lives and was particularly concerned with physical and mental health issues. For example, in 2012 it consulted with physicians at the Johns Hopkins School of Medicine, Columbia University School of Public Health, Boston's Children's Hospital, and other health organizations, with the intention of developing a coordinated approach to deal with the unique health care needs of adolescent and young adult males. Several of the project goals included identifying effective interventions, creating prevention checklists and guidelines, and promoting public policies that supported the proposed clinical guidelines. This initiative focused on sexual and reproductive health issues for young men, but it did not deal directly with fathering per se. Nevertheless, this type of organization could still indirectly help prepare men to be health conscious fathers who are attentive to both their own and their children's health and fitness needs.

Some of the strategies I've advocated over the years to help boys develop a stronger caregiving approach toward children are quite similar to what should be done to encourage young men to monitor their own health and fitness more carefully.[7] Boys need to be taught to become more self-aware in the present and inspired to imagine what kind of father they want to be in the future.

Another critical step in getting boys and young men to make smarter personal decisions is to capitalize on the remarkable leverage male peer groups often wield. Typically, peer pressure is perceived as being negative, but is it possible to harness this social energy in a positive way? In some respects, the distinction between peer pressure and support may not always be clear. Whether it is school activities and athletics, mentoring programs, recreational leagues, or community youth initiatives, one way to help young males become more mindful about maintaining good health is to convince them that their high-status male peers endorse a program's health-based mission. Part of the trick, of course, is to get the high-status guys to buy in to messages that reject drug use, smoking, drinking and driving, irresponsible treatment of head trauma, and risky sexual practices while embracing others that promote healthy eating, sunscreen use, regular exercise, safer sex practices, and the respectful treatment of girls and women.

The power of peer pressure or support doesn't end with young men; it can influence how adult men orient themselves to their bodies and health. When friends tell friends they've had a colonoscopy, prostate exam, or just an annual checkup they let their friends know—directly or indirectly— that it's a good idea to reach out to the medical community for health assessments. Friends can also challenge one another to alter their self-destructive habits or to just become a bit more health conscious in their diet and exercise.

For example, in chapter 4 I described how a powerful message delivered to Owen, a very overweight former paratrooper, transformed his life. Hearing another man candidly tell him that he was going to die prematurely and leave his wife and kids without a husband and father became a turning point for Owen. He was forced to think about how his poor health habits— culminating in his eventual death—would impact his family. Although it is unusual for fathers to undergo Owen's type of dramatic makeover from being a grossly obese, lethargic man to a slim, energetic yoga devotee, plenty of other fathers describe how they adopted a healthier lifestyle once they began to take their fatherhood responsibilities more seriously.

It can be challenging to get unhealthy men and fathers—some who have grown accustomed to their negative routines over many years—to alter their lifestyles. Men's circumstances are too diverse for a one-size-fits-all approach to convince men to change their perspective on their personal health or to get them more invested in their children's health and fitness. However, finding creative ways to alter workplace cultures and secure social support from peers and family members is surely a step in the right direction.

Perhaps the most propitious time to get men's attention is when they are expecting their first child. Although first-time fathers-in-waiting include a wide range of teenagers, young adult men, and, increasingly, men in their thirties and even forties, most are excited and nervous about their new experience. Some enter this new life stage with solid health insurance and are dialed in to good health practices for themselves as well as their children. Others are burdened with inadequate or no health care coverage and beleaguered by poor health habits, some of which are likely to produce ill effects for their children over time. Although social initiatives can benefit all fathers, they are particularly needed for the latter subset.

My call for men to adopt a more health conscious approach to life for themselves and their children is tempered by the need for a more critical vision of what health represents and the ideology that increasingly frames how individuals relate to it in the United States. If men accept the challenge and heighten their sensitivity to health issues they should also consider how their choices are shaped by a health rhetoric with moralistic overtones. That rhetoric often leads observers to judge people negatively who engage in behaviors such as cigarette smoking or eating junk food or exhibit conditions such as persistent coughing or obesity that are perceived to be unhealthy. Others tend to see those being judged as lacking sufficient character, will, or sound moral judgment to make healthier choices. Thus, as fathers pay more attention to health and fitness concerns for themselves and others, they can deepen their self-awareness by understanding how their preferences and choices influence their reactions to others.

In the Internet age we can easily inundate ourselves with scientific findings and all sorts of competing expert advice about what is or isn't good for us in terms of diet, supplements, exercise, addictions, risk taking, therapy, surgeries, and more. To complicate matters, these messages are often revised over time, sometimes in dramatic fashion. Sorting through and making sense of this information is challenging, time-consuming, and often frustrating. Although I've advocated basic health- and fitness-related themes in this book (regular exercise, avoiding substance abuse, honoring concussion protocol, regular visits to a doctor, sunblock use, helmet use), dads can make a range of choices and still believe they are practicing a conscientious, healthy lifestyle while simultaneously promoting similarly good choices for their children. I recognize that trying to make a definitive statement about what is healthy behavior is fraught with difficulty. For example, not all dads will have the free time, desire, or resources to adopt a diet and exercise regimen similar to mine, but many can still experience relatively good health. At the same time, I believe fathers in general need to be more attentive to their own and their children's health and fitness and willing to take meaningful steps to improve both—at the very least, on their own terms. A first step toward that goal is for them to make a conscious effort to learn more about the human body and the kinds of things that can affect its functioning.

Ironically, for dads intensely focused on their health, body, fitness, and physical performance, concerns about balancing personal and family time can taint the virtues of pursuing a healthy lifestyle. Can too much of a good thing be bad for family relations and children's well-being? Perhaps. When fathers train extensively for marathons, triathlons, and other endurance events it typically limits their time with their families. Although some endurance athletes try to coordinate their training to minimize their time away from their children and partners, the rigorous training circumstances that often define endurance athletes' lives restrict how involved they can be with their children.[8] As a result, unless these dads frequently incorporate their children into their workouts they tend to miss out on chances to be more directly involved in monitoring their children's health and fitness. So the children are exposed to a parental role model for fitness, but it can come at a cost: fathers will be less available to mentor their children directly.

Although it is important to consider how people perceive good health and navigate their route to achieve it—for themselves as well as their children—we must also recognize how the stark realities of social class affect many dads' experiences in the health matrix. For sure, challenging dads to become more health conscious for themselves and their children is a vital part of a father-friendly social change agenda. However, attempts to inspire must be supplemented with practical strategies to help dads who have the desire but not the money to ensure their children are exposed to healthy options. Poor dads, many living in disadvantaged neighborhoods, struggle to provide certain types of health and fitness options for their children. For these fathers and their families, city planners, churches, schools, public health organizations, and other community groups can offer support. They can empower the poor dads who are emotionally invested in their children to circumvent the everyday barriers that limit their ability to make a more meaningful difference in their health and fitness. For example, city officials can devote more resources to develop family-friendly recreational facilities and keep them safe. They can also create business zone policies that will attract supermarket chains and health food stores. So too, various types of organizations can reduce or waive registration and equipment fees for poor families and dads who want to enroll their children in community- or school-based youth sports programs.

TRANSITIONING TO BEING A DAD

In the months leading up to a birth (especially a first birth) and immediately following it, obstetricians, pediatricians, nurses, parent educators, and others can do more to encourage men to focus on their health and their child's health. In chapter 2, I highlighted how the health care community has made considerable strides over the past fifty or so years to incorporate men more fully into the prenatal and childbirth process. Research shows that getting men more involved in their partner's pregnancy leads to better outcomes for mom and child. The next step is to turn prospective and new fathers' attention toward their own health and to compel them to be more active in attending to their children's health and fitness needs as well.

One practical challenge is to entice men to improve their orientation toward health and fitness without alienating them. Despite various efforts to make men more central to the process of pregnancy and birth, men are still seen as secondary players in the procreative realm. Pregnant women are cared for by obstetricians who rightfully see them, and in some respect the fetuses, as their patients. Women are regularly encouraged to be mindful of their health and to eat well, exercise and rest in a responsible way, take supplements, and avoid harmful substances. Similarly, childbirth educators and midwives typically focus on the mother as the primary recipient of their message while talking to men as coaches and helpers. Meanwhile, prospective fathers' states of physical or mental health are seldom if ever addressed or questioned. Even programs like Baby Boot Camp do not systematically address men's own health status; rather, they attempt to instill soon-to-be fathers with more confidence about the important role they can play in caring for their children. The program attempts to establish and polish men's caregiving skill set without challenging men to improve their own self-care.

Prenatal sessions and fatherhood workshops need to be expanded to educate fathers about how their lifestyle habits related to health and fitness can influence their children's well-being. No doubt, some soon-to-be fathers will resist any assertive attempt to assess and alter their health-related behaviors. Nonetheless, health promotion initiatives that target these men may prove to be instrumental in changing the cycle of poor health behaviors and outcomes that fathers can pass on to their children.

Once a child is born, it is commonplace for a pediatrician, and sometimes a lactation consultant, to join the mix of health care providers who monitor the baby, and to lesser extent the mother. The pediatricians I spoke with, as well as the ones described to me, typically do not ask about the fathers' health-related habits, such as diet or exercise. About the most they or their assistants do is to ask whether anyone in the house smokes as part of the standard new-patient-history that is obtained on behalf of an infant or older child. When children exhibit particular health issues like asthma, drinking, or diabetes, pediatricians may ask additional questions about family members to get a better sense of the family diet, smoking, or alcohol consumption patterns. Occasionally, pediatricians may even confront parents about their habits if they feel they will exacerbate children's already compromised health.

Yet some pediatricians make it their business to encourage fathers from the outset to be more attentive to their infant's needs whether they are completely healthy or struggling in some way. Craig Garfield, the Chicago-based pediatrician discussed in chapter 6, is quite active in this regard. He is committed to reaching out to dads during that first day or two when they're with their newborns in the hospital. Garfield sees this period as a teachable moment, so he capitalizes on dads' euphoria and implores them to acquire hands-on caregiving experience. He also shares with them concrete strategies that enable them to be a supportive partner to their breast-feeding partner. In the hospital and during the initial well-baby visits Garfield strives to be as "explicit" as possible with the dads.[9] Mimicking one of his typical conversations with a dad, Garfield illustrates:

> "Here's what you can do for breastfeeding, when she's gonna breastfeed make sure she has the pillows in place that will get the baby right at the level of the breast to do like A, B, and C with the baby so it gets a good shot, make sure she has something to drink, change the diaper, help her kind of relax the shoulders, make sure she's not all hunched up that's gonna stop the milk flow." And I feel like, once you start talking to these dads they like, their eyes open they get fully engaged and are listening to what you are saying.

Speaking on behalf of most pediatricians, Garfield notes that during the initial office visits, doctors often find it difficult to have extensive conversations about father involvement. Most doctors are pressed for time when they see their patients. This limited time frame can also help discourage pediatricians from exploring how parents manage their own health and fitness. Despite the restricted time frame of the well-baby visit, Garfield believes it is critical to encourage the "mom to let the father be involved and learn from that involvement." From his perspective, this is essential to help fathers develop a connection with their newborn. When he turns his attention to dads during the newborn period he tells them that they should "get in early and get in often, you know, learn how you want to soothe your baby, how you want to diaper your baby, how you want to talk to and sing to your baby, and [that] stuff is really important."

Some states and communities sponsor well-baby programs that send health care professionals out to homes to check on infants and their parents. While some programs are designed to deal with premature infants or other young children with serious health issues, some initiatives include both healthy and health-compromised kids. Most of these initiatives are designed as prevention programs to ensure the health and well-being of women, children, and their families.

Thomas, the pediatrician, was once involved with a home-visiting program in New England that sought to engage fathers. That initiative tried to arrange evening visits to increase the chances of including fathers, but the staff found it challenging because doing night-time visits was not always safe in some neighborhoods. Thomas supports these home-visiting programs in principle but acknowledges that they tend to pop up in different places for a while but do not last. "I often see short-term initiatives that don't end up being sustained, either they're grant funded or they're, someone takes the lead and that person gets tired and moves on, they kind of tend to dwindle. So I haven't seen real sustained things."

Unfortunately, in the United States, the political will is lacking to fund adequately home-based outreach programs that could help all new parents create a healthy environment for their young children. A 2011 report sponsored by the nonprofit organization Pew Charitable Trusts (Pew) indicates that forty-six states provided funds for early childhood home visiting activities, with many of these efforts targeting at-risk families.[10] Among the participating states, at least thirty-four reported investing in at least two prenatal and early childhood home visiting programs. Twenty-one states funded three or more programs. Pew's analysis of survey data shows that programs did not "consistently target at-risk families and none had the funding or infrastructure to reach all the high-risk families."

One notable program, Healthy Families Massachusetts, is seen as innovative in the field because it began in 2001 to develop the means to collect and analyze data to evaluate its performance. A statewide initiative serving roughly three thousand families with a first-time parent under age twenty-one, HFM is supported by the Children's Trust and is funded through the federal Maternal, Infant, and Early Childhood Home Visiting program (MIECHV). The 2015 Children's Trust Strengthening Families annual report highlights its Fatherhood Initiative, including the Fathers and Family Network, which provides "extensive training and technical assistance on strategies for working with fathers and co-parents."[11]

In principle, home visiting programs could be tailored to monitor the mother's and the father's overall health. For decades, researchers have been pointing out that mothers' postpartum depression is a pervasive and serious problem that affects how well mothers care for their children.[12] Children are more likely to experience a wide range of emotional, psychological, and behavioral difficulties when their mothers suffer from depression. In contrast, much less is known about fathers' prenatal and postpartum depression.[13] A review of forty-three studies suggests that about 10 percent of fathers experience prenatal and postpartum depression.[14] In one large study of fathers in the United Kingdom roughly 4 percent report depression eight weeks after the birth of their baby. Among the UK fathers, those who report in this way tend to have children who exhibit more behavioral problems when they are between three and five years of age.[15] This finding holds when the mother's level of depression is controlled, and the pattern is stronger for boys than in girls. The authors speculate that fathers may affect them directly because the depressed fathers may provide poorer child care, or indirectly because fathers who suffer from emotional problems are less supportive of the mothers of the children.

A small but increasingly vocal cadre of pediatricians in the United States is trying to lobby their peers to recognize that just like mothers, fathers can also experience emotional and mental difficulties after their child is born. However, the effort to promote screenings for fathers as well as mothers has been an uphill battle. Only recently has the medical community slowly begun to recognize that some men experience a kind of postpartum depression. One pediatrician in my study, serving on a state legislative commission, repeatedly suggests that "we should be screening fathers as well as mothers, and that one of the ways in which fathers matter is not necessarily just with sadness or weepiness or, some typical signs of depression, but drinking, drug abuse, withdrawal, and domestic abuse."

David Hill, a pediatrician-dad and the author of *Dad to Dad: Parenting Like a Pro*, is another avant-garde medical professional who is helping to transform the health matrix so that fathers feel more welcome and eager to participate in their children's care.[16] The practical tips Dr. Hill presents about infant and child development, baby basics (crying, sleeping, pooping, and eating), vaccines, and more offer dads valuable insights they can use to nurture their children. His approach also reminds pediatricians that they need to step up and reassure dads that baby and child care are opportunities they should embrace without apprehension.

DISCOVERING DADS IN THE HEALTH MATRIX

The need for programmatic help is especially relevant to those dads whose health is compromised or who have children managing special needs. More than half of the fathers I interviewed fell into one of these two categories. Although several fathers received assistance from health-related initiatives that targeted the specific disability that affected their family, most dealt with their circumstances while relying on standard consultations with medical professionals and treatment protocols. To date, the bulk of whatever attention fathers have received from the health care system has been from those whose primary interest is children's well-being—those with or without special needs.

For more than a decade, some health care professionals have called for their peers to be more attentive in their clinical work to how fathers can make significant contributions to their children with or without special needs. These professionals have tried to revamp how their colleagues perceive and respond to fathers in their clinical work. In their 2003 essay "Promoting Father-Friendly Healthcare," Linda Tiedje and Cynthia Darling-Fisher challenged health care organizations and professionals to do a self-assessment of how they interact with fathers.[17] They implicitly sought to strengthen the partnership between fathers and health care professionals by encouraging their professional peers to consider the extent to which and how they acknowledge the father's presence, manage their body language, make eye contact with the father, ask information of and give information to fathers, and have developed beliefs about fathers' role in health care settings based on their own personal experience with family and friends of fathers' involvement in these areas. In addition, the Texas Department of Health Services developed a useful worksheet that provides doctors with guidance on how to create a more inclusive environment for dads in the special supplemental nutrition program WIC (Women, Infants, and Children), and it created a worksheet for medical staff to assess whether a doctor's office is "father friendly."[18]

Several of the pediatric health care professionals I spoke with explicitly mention their conscious efforts to draw fathers into a dialogue about their child by directing questions to them and making eye contact. I sensed, though, that these professionals are quite conscious of the time crunch they are under when doing their consultations, so even if they want to incorporate a father into the consultation more fully, they may be reluctant to devote too much time to those efforts if the father does not appear to be a key informant for his child's health history and immediate condition.

With rates of autism in the United States on the rise, targeted efforts to help fathers of children with autism become more effective caregivers are clearly warranted. One team of researchers discovered that it's possible to implement an in-home training program designed to teach fathers four caregiving skills (imitating with animation, expectant waiting, following the child's lead, and commenting on the child) that parents can use to generate social reciprocity with their children who have autism.[19] The training showed that fathers can learn and use these skills effectively and can be taught how to train mothers to use the same set of interpersonal skills.

This program and similar ones yet to be developed for children with other chronic conditions can encourage fathers to be more proactive and develop their confidence when interacting with their children with special needs. These efforts may need to be tailored to the unique features of specific ailments including but not limited to Down syndrome, diabetes, blindness, cerebral palsy, and paralysis.

INITIATIVES TO PROMOTE HEALTH- AND FITNESS-CONSCIOUS FATHERING

Most recent organized efforts to promote good fathering in the United States and other Western countries assume that if fathers spend more quality time with their children it will lead to better behavioral, cognitive, emotional, psychological, and social outcomes for the children. Interventions address diverse issues, including fathers' work skills and self-sufficiency, the level and quality of father-child interactions, healthy couple relationships and coparenting, recidivism, mental health and psychological well-being, and risky behaviors such as unsafe sex, substance abuse, and crime.[20] Unfortunately, despite the surge in new fatherhood programs during the past few decades, relatively little is known about how fatherhood programming influences fathers' relationships with their children or child outcomes.[21] Although some interventions focus on health concerns more directly than others, most fatherhood programs can produce potential health benefits for fathers, children, and families.

In terms of ideology, we need to transform once and for all the outdated stereotype of the father as the exclusive or even primary breadwinner. Instead, we need to embrace in everyday life and in our policies and programs the idea that a father should be attentive to and nurture his children in addition to contributing directly or indirectly to a parenting arrangement that financially supports them.[22] In other words, he should be free to be a stay-at-home dad or work part-time if his partner is open to supporting the family financially. But even if he assumes a primary breadwinning role, he should commit himself to being as responsive as possible to his children's needs—including those involving health and fitness.

By focusing on the health matrix specifically, a recasting of fatherhood responsibilities can best be realized if stakeholders address personal, organizational, and cultural forces that affect how men are oriented toward their own and their children's health, fitness, and well-being. Initiatives that foster opportunities for dads to develop a nurturing approach to fathering can encourage them to be more proactive in guiding their children's specific health and fitness choices.

A pervasive theme running through many of the fatherhood interventions is that getting men to care for themselves is a critical step toward getting them to be attentive and responsible fathers.[23] This message is keenly relevant to the lifestyle decisions men make that influence their health and fitness. We must do a better job of getting men to understand more fully, and as soon as possible, that their everyday habits involving diet, exercise, risk taking, sleep and relaxation, and substance use not only affect them but can leave a lasting impression on their children as well. In addition to helping men see the connection between their actions and outcomes for their children, social initiatives need to help men make lifestyle changes that will improve their lives and enable them to model healthy habits for their children. Ideally, more men will adopt healthier practices before a child is conceived or at least before the child is born.

The ultimate goal—to transform men's thinking and behavior in ways that make men personally more health conscious and intimately invested in their children's health and fitness—is no easy task. It can be accomplished best by generating a wide range of collaborative partnerships between individuals and community groups. Efforts that enhance the four partnerships I emphasize (father-child, father-coparent, father-nonfamily members, and community organizations' interactions) can help fathers navigate the health matrix more productively for themselves and their children. This perspective reminds us that good fathering extends well beyond establishing healthy family rituals and habits in the home. It also entails the subtle as well as focused exchanges with others in the community that build connections and opportunities that enhance kids' lives.

Some partnerships require leaders from health care organizations, community agencies, and state and federal governments to prioritize the contributions fathers can make to enhance children's health and fitness. Yet individual men are not helpless. They can take practical steps to alter their own lives and their relationships with their children. Of course, some men are better situated than others to make things happen. Some are constrained because they have health problems, financial difficulties, limited access to community recreation sites, demanding and inflexible jobs, or live apart from their children. Children bring their own set of characteristics such as age, personality, athletic aptitude, and special needs status that can affect fathers' opportunities to make a difference. Family circumstances, including the number of children and the mother's disposition, will influence fathers' options as well. Although fathers' personal and family diversity preclude outlining a standard set of recommendations that can apply ideally across the board, some general suggestions for what fathers can do themselves include the following approaches:

- Be responsive to hands-on infant care (for example, diapering, bathing, administering medicine) and sleep and feeding schedules.
- Attend and be active in prenatal workshops and well-baby checkups.
- Take the initiative to place children in organized physical activities including recreational community youth leagues.
- Provide practical and emotional support to children's sports activities and volunteer to coach.
- Commit to doing regular physical activity and exercise with children outdoors at playgrounds and in nature, and at home or other indoor facilities.
- Develop food purchasing and preparation rituals that include label reviewing, nutrition talks, ventures to grocery stores and farmers' markets, downloading and executing recipes.
- Create a home environment that accentuates health and a lifestyle that promotes fitness (for example, healthy food choices, gardening, jungle gym equipment for the yard, outside and inside sports equipment, health/sports magazines).
- Teach kids skills that will allow them to feel comfortable exercising.

- Use technology (for example, BabyBump, Fooducate, yoga Wii, cycle computers, apps that count calories) to encourage children's goal-oriented fitness activities.
- Attend pediatrician visits regularly and help monitor children's medications and therapies.
- Act as a health advocate for children in specific ways when interacting with persons in the community who monitor them (for example, coaches and concussions, school teachers and snacks, youth ministers and fitness options).
- Invest in one's own health by engaging in regular physical activity, eating well, and avoiding risk-taking behaviors.
- Model a healthy approach to managing emotions and displays of masculinity.

Although few men are truly helpless to alter at least some of their health-related habits, some clearly need support from friends and family to change their unhealthy outlook and practices. Others need help sustaining the healthy lifestyle they have adopted already. As children age, they can play a more active role in motivating their fathers, as well as their mothers, to think differently about their health and fitness. By what they say and do, children can reinforce some of my specific suggestions that target men.

How can we design social initiatives to mobilize kids to help their dads? Once again, productive partnerships between community groups and families are vital. School-based and public health programs can be implemented separately or collaboratively. They can offer kids creative opportunities to encourage fathers to become more health conscious as well as entice them to try healthy activities with them. I've organized an entire section, "Teachers' Corner," on my *Dads & Kids: Health & Fitness Talk* website to provide teachers with assignment options for students of different ages. For example, teachers in health and home economics classes who talk to kids about nutrition and healthy food options can use my templates or develop their own exercises that place kids into conversations with their fathers and mothers. Kids with a father figure in their lives might work on joint projects related to food production, grocery shopping, or meal preparation. I was impressed listening to several dads talk about their homeschooling efforts to integrate educational lessons into real-life activities at the grocery store and in the kitchen.

Activities can be developed to encourage fathers to come to school during the school day, aftercare, or on a weekend to participate in some sort of event promoting healthy living. Public health departments can partner with schools on specific initiatives. Imagine a hands-on cooking program that offers middle and high school students the chance to learn alongside their parents about healthy ways to cook. Similarly, fitness clubs and large child care facilities can sponsor outdoor or indoor family fitness events that provide children and their dads and moms an opportunity to play certain games, test their athletic skills, and have different screenings done (such as those for hearing, vision, and blood pressure).

For several years I've taken Phoenix to an afternoon event sponsored by a gym I belong to, Gainesville Health and Fitness Center (GHFC), which offers family members a chance to: run an obstacle course, try different tasks with athletic balls, do pushups, run races, have their vertical jump measured, and more. Participating in this annual event has solidified our joint commitment to spending time together doing fitness activities. Although I was the one who pulled Phoenix into the GHFC event, public initiatives can also stress the value of community organizations targeting kids to help them reach out to their fathers in order to experience the health matrix in a more proactive, productive way.

THE FUTURE

I wrote this book during a propitious moment in American history, with public debate about health care never more passionate and pervasive. The debate has often dealt with the administrative side of managing and implementing health care reform, with some commentary targeting the ideological principles that support or oppose the Affordable Care Act. Beyond the health wars waged by conservatives and liberals, and the federal government's implementation of what is often called Obamacare, popular culture is awash with books, articles, news sound bites, and commercials relevant to the worlds of health and fitness. Many of the messages point to research findings, human interest stories, policy and program updates, the virtues of alternative health care modalities such as acupuncture, biofeedback, massage therapy, meditation, and yoga, or commercial products and services designed to improve emotional, mental, physical, and spiritual health.

Americans are repeatedly reminded of the latest diet fads and sometimes told of the dangers of risky behaviors like drinking while pregnant, drinking and driving, driving without a seatbelt, driving and texting, smoking, and unprotected sex. They hear that exercise can reduce risks of cardiovascular disease and bring other benefits to their quality of life. They learn about the most recent food supplement or derivative that will expunge whatever ails them. Unfortunately, because contradictory messages about nutrition and diets are common and conventional wisdom about these matters is often revised in response to the latest research, individuals are often befuddled about what they should do to live a healthy life.

Ironically, while Americans are increasingly exposed to messages about the value of remaining healthy and fit they are also bombarded at a record rate by commercial efforts to have them consume food and beverages in ways not in their long-term best interests. In recent decades, the commercialized American diet built on fast-food staples like burgers, fries, pizza, wings, fried chicken, and super-sized sugary sodas has helped to exacerbate health problems for adults and youth alike. For many, this unhealthy diet has become the norm. Even health-conscious parents must confront the appeal it has for their children, who are often pressured by peers to eat this way. Youth who watch sports on TV are also inundated with creative, alluring ads for beer and other alcohol products. Even though commercials avoid representing middle school or high school youth, young people get the message that drinking goes hand-in-hand with being cool and having a fun time hanging out with friends.

In the end, we are left with too many sobering health trends in the form of high rates of obesity, eating disorders, binge drinking, alcoholism, drug addiction, suicide, infant mortality, and a range of diseases, like diabetes, that are at least partially influenced by lifestyle choices for some individuals. These patterns compromise the chances for many fathers, mothers, and kids to maximize the quality of their health in the short- and long-term.

As political battles continue over how best to handle rising health care costs, we must confront the reality that many of our health problems as a society are self-inflicted. Accounting for the expanding challenges of caring for an aging population, rising health care costs are in no small measure the result of our failure to encourage and enable individuals to live healthier lives when they are younger. The prevention ethos, while a trendy notion in some circles, is too often overlooked or ignored when public institutions conduct their everyday business.

Unfortunately, I am frustrated by this reality when teachers and after-school staff make junk food and candy readily available to my son and his classmates. Cultural tolerance for how institutions interact with our children has changed considerably in recent decades. We are more vigilant than ever about stranger danger and we more closely monitor teachers being alone with or hugging children, yet we are seemingly open to those same teachers and caregivers supplying our children with candy rewards for school performance and attendance.[24] Perhaps my memory is faulty, but I cannot recall ever receiving candy rewards from teachers for doing my schoolwork.

Lost within this mass of activity are concerns about how dads from varying backgrounds affect and are affected by the health matrix that includes their kids. By talking to an eclectic sample of dads and focusing on them as men, I highlight the value of treating dads as central players in the health matrix involving young people—from babies to young adults. Fathers can be relevant in social settings whether they are in good health or face their own chronic health problems. Likewise, efforts should be directed toward helping men become nurturing dads whether they have healthy kids or children with special needs. Ideally, we must continue to revamp policies and practices in work, health care, education, and other settings in order to build upon the emerging trend for dads to be more nurturing irrespective of their level of commitment to their paid work.

Moving forward, we need to frame health as not simply a physical, emotional, or mental attribute expressed by a particular person such as a child or father. Instead, we need to see that health has a social, interpersonal quality. In some respects, a man's health is a negotiated experience. A man develops a sense of his health and fitness through his interactions with different types of social networks including family, friends, and health care professionals.[25] Similarly, youth develop their orientation toward health and fitness through their interactions with and observations of others, including their fathers.

This view is consistent with the idea that nurturing dads are sensitive to, and engaged with, the various people who make up the larger social fabric that influences their children's lives—whether those people are part of the family, extended family, neighborhood, or community organizations. Even though health and fitness are not the only issues of concern to nurturing dads, they represent critical ones, especially for men who have serious health conditions or have children with special needs. Ideally, encouraging dads to become more nurturing will nudge them to become more health conscious for themselves and their children.

The cultural messages about children's health that dominate the health care industry and popular culture are tailored disproportionately toward mothers.[26] Over the years, the gendered division of labor has made it seem natural to target moms because they typically have been the primary caregivers for children and the ones most likely to provide detailed health histories for them. On balance, moms still are more likely to be the primary caregivers and they are therefore better than dads in providing health histories for children. But we are in the midst of a protracted shift in how moms and dads define their identities in relation to paid work and home life.

If we are serious about the ideals that define a profeminist agenda, we must recast how dads fit into the family health matrix and social institutions must provide them better incentives and the practical means to be nurturing parents. Our society will be a lot better off when men, and the general public, recognize that "good fathering" demands that dads be proactive in doing all they can to enhance their own health and fitness while doing the same for their children.

NOTES

CHAPTER 1 MAPPING DADS' PLACE IN THE HEALTH MATRIX

1. William Marsiglio, "Healthy Dads, Healthy Kids," *Contexts* 8 (2009): 22–27.
2. Fiola J. Moola, "This Is the Best Fatal Illness That You Can Have: Contrasting and Comparing the Experiences of Parenting Youth with Cystic Fibrosis and Congenital Heart Disease," *Qualitative Health Research* 22 (2012): 212–225.
3. Jennifer Newbould, Felicity Smith, and Sally-Anne Francis, "'I'm Fine Doing It on My Own': Partnership between Young People and Their Parents in the Management of Medication for Asthma and Diabetes," *Journal of Child Health Care* 12 (2008): 116–128.
4. Moola, "This Is the Best Fatal Illness That You Can Have"; André Samson et al., "The Lived Experience of Hope among Parents of a Child with Duchenne Muscular Dystrophy: Perceiving the Human Being Beyond the Illness," *Chronic Illness* 5 (2009): 103–114; Jane Ware and Hitesh Raval, "A Qualitative Investigation of Fathers' Experiences of Looking After a Child with a Life-limiting Illness, in Process and Retrospect," *Clinical Child Psychology and Psychiatry* 12 (2007): 549–565.
5. World Health Organization, http://www.who.int/about/en/, accessed February 14, 2016.
6. Jonathan M. Metzl, "Why 'Against Health'?" in *Against Health: How Health Became the New Morality*, ed. Jonathan M. Mentz and Anna Kirland (New York: New York University Press, 2010), 1–2; see also Jonathan M. Metzl and Anna Kirland, eds., *Against Health: How Health Became the New Morality* (New York: New York University Press, 2010). This edited volume presents a diverse set of chapters that explore alternative visions of what constitutes health. In presenting a critical interpretation of health, the volume examines how various social and political forces shape the ways health has become a complex and socially constructed reality with significant moral overtones.
7. Metzl, "Why 'Against Health'?"
8. Adams et al., "Overweight, Obesity, and Mortality in a Large Prospective Cohort of Persons 50 to 71 Years Old," *New England Journal of Medicine* 355(8) (2006): 763–778; Donald A. Barr, *Health Disparities in the United States: Social Class, Race, Ethnicity, and Health* (Baltimore: Johns Hopkins University Press, 2008).
9. Joe Kelly, *Dads and Daughters: How to Inspire, Understand, and Support Your Daughter When She's Growing Up So Fast* (New York: Broadway Books, 2002); Linda Nielsen, *Father-Daughter Relationships: Contemporary Research and Issues* (New York: Routledge, 2012).
10. This project initially began with me training several students to use a semi-structured interview guide I created to conduct pilot interviews with twelve fathers in

Gainesville and Miami, Florida, between February 2008 and March 2010. I then personally conducted the remaining seventy-five interviews with fathers and fifteen interviews
with pediatric health care professionals between April 2012 and September 2013.

11. William L. Coleman and Craig Garfield, and American Academy of Pediatrics,
Committee on Psychosocial Aspects of Child and Family Health, "Fathers and Pediatricians: Enhancing Men's Roles in the Care and Development of Their Children," *Pediatrics* 113, no. 5 (2004): 1406–1411.

12. William Marsiglio, "Being a Dad, Studying Fathers: Personal Reflections," in *Papa,
PhD: Essays on Fatherhood by Men in the Academy*, ed. Mary Ruth Marotte, Paige Martin
Reynolds, and Ralph James Savarese (New Brunswick, NJ: Rutgers University Press,
2011), 135–140.

13. Dr. Axe, "Stop Using Canola Oil Immediately," http://draxe.com/canola-oil-gm/.

14. Center for Disease Control and Prevention, "Early Release of Selected Estimates
Based on Data from the 2014 National Health Interview Survey," data table for figure 7.2. Percentage of adults aged eighteen and over who met the 2008 federal physical activity guidelines for aerobic activity through leisure-time aerobic activity, by age
group and sex: United States, 2014. http://www.cdc.gov/nchs/data/nhis/earlyrelease/
earlyrelease201409_07.pdf, accessed May 18, 2015.

15. Diana T. Cohen, *Iron Dads: Managing Work, Family, and Endurance Sport Identities*
(New Brunswick, NJ: Rutgers University Press, 2016); Anne M. Gardner, "Triathletes,
40-Somethings, Going for Youth," *New York Times*, October 24, 2010, http://www
.nytimes.com/2010/10/24/fashion/24triathlon.html?pagewanted=all, accessed September 21, 2102.

16. Eric Anderson and Edward Kian, "Examining Media Contestation of Masculinity
and Head Trauma in the National Football League," *Men and Masculinities* 15 (2012):
152–173.

17. Ken Belson, "N.F.L. Agrees to Settle Concussion Suit for $765 Million," *New York
Times*, August 29, 2013, http://www.nytimes.com/2013/08/30/sports/football/judge
-announces-settlement-in-nfl-concussion-suit.html?pagewanted=all, accessed September 14, 2013.

18. Steven C. Marcus and Mark Olfson, "National Trends in the Treatment for Depression from 1998 to 2007," *Archives of General Psychiatry* 67 (2010): 1265–1273.

19. Laura Landro, "New Ads Try to Shock Men Into Going to See the Doctor,"
The Wall Street Journal, June 15, 2010, http://online.wsj.com/article/SB100014240
52748704463504575301130174214118.html, accessed February 14, 2016.

20. Center for Disease Control and Prevention, "Table 88 (page 1 of 3). Visits to Physician Offices, Hospital Outpatient Departments, and Hospital Emergency Departments,
by Age, Sex, and Race: United States, selected years 1995–2011," http://www.cdc.gov/
nchs/hus/contents2012.htm#088, accessed February 14, 2016.

21. "ESPN Campaign Urges Men to Seek Preventive Health Care," *New York Times*,
May 5, 2008, http://www.nytimes.com/2008/05/05/business/media/05adnewsletter
.html?_r=1%26ref=login%26pagewanted=print, accessed September 14, 2013.

22. Landro, "New Ads Try to Shock Men Into Going to See the Doctor."

23. Abbvie, http://www.driveforfive.com/, accessed February 14, 2016.

24. Audit Bureau of Circulation. The totals represent circulation averages for six months ending on June 30, 2012, http://abcas3.accessabc.com/ecirc/magtitlesearch .asp, accessed October 4, 2012.

25. Emily Senay and Rob Waters, *From Boys to Men: A Women's Guide to the Health of Husbands, Partners, Sons, Fathers, and Brothers* (New York: Scribner, 2004). This book underscores the gender gap in how men and women approach health care, focusing on strategies women can use to do a better job of helping their male loved ones manage their health productively. I draw attention to how men can and do develop better self-care philosophies.

26. David Wilkins and Erick Savoye, *Men's Health Around the World: A Review of Policy and Progress Across 11 Countries*, 2009, http://www.raf.mod.uk/community/mura-raf -community/assets/File/Mens%20Health%20Around%20the%20World.pdf, accessed September 18, 2015.

27. Ibid. See also Noel Richardson and Paula Carroll, for a report on Ireland in 2008, http://www.mhfi.org/menshealthpolicy.pdf, accessed September 18, 2015.

28. United Nations, *Men in Families and Family Policy in a Changing World* (2011), http://www.un.org/esa/socdev/family/docs/men-in-families.pdf, accessed October 19, 2012.

29. Ibid., 33.

30. http://www.men-care.org/Who-We-Are/About-Us.aspx, accessed September 26, 2013.

31. Men's Health Braintrust/Dialogue on Men's Health, A Framework for Advancing the Overall Health and Wellness of America's Boys and Men, 2012, http://www .menshealthnetwork.org/library/Dialogue1.pdf, accessed February 1, 2016.

32. A notable exception is the Australian-based Healthy Dads, Healthy Kids community intervention program designed to target overweight fathers. See Morgan et al., 2014. "The 'Healthy Dads, Healthy Kids' Community Randomized Controlled Trial: A Community-Based Healthy Lifestyle Program for Fathers and Their Children." *Preventive Medicine* 61 (2014): 90–99. The intervention "motivated fathers to engage in physical activity with their children and involve them in healthy eating opportunities. In turn, the children were encouraged to prompt and encourage their fathers to adopt healthier behaviors. This reciprocal reinforcement of healthier behaviors between father and child(ren) was targeted in the program and is particularly pertinent when adopting and refining behaviors" (95). The program reports improved health outcomes for both fathers and their primary school-aged children. In addition, Coffield and colleagues, in "Shape Up Somerville: Change in Parent Body Mass Indexes during a Child-Targeted, Community-Based Environmental Change Intervention," *American Journal of Public Health* 105, no. 2 (2015): E83–389, report promising findings from their nonrandomized control study of a program, Shape Up Somerville, that targeted children's obesity in thirty elementary schools in Massachusetts communities. The child-centered intervention resulted in reduced BMI values for the children's parents.

33. Jeffrey Levi et al., *The State of Obesity Report: Better Policies for a Healthier American 2014*, Trust for America's Health, 2014, Robert Wood Johnson Foundation, http://www .rwjf.org/content/dam/farm/reports/reports/2014/rwjf414829, accessed May 19, 2015.

34. Josephine Fraser et al., "Paternal Influences on Children's Weight Gain: A Systematic Review," *Fathering* 9 (2011): 252–267.

35. Sinead Brophy et al., "Child Fitness and Father's BMI are Important Factors in Childhood Obesity: A School Based Cross-sectional Study," *Plosone* 7, no. 5 (2012): e36597: 1–7; E. Freeman et al., "Preventing and Treating Childhood Obesity: Time to Target Fathers," *International Journal of Obesity* 36 (2012): 12–15.

36. Data from the CDC's *Morbidity and Mortality Weekly Report*, November 28, 2014.

37. Stephan E. Gilman et al., "Parental Smoking and Adolescent Smoking Initiation: An Intergenerational Perspective on Tobacco Control," *Pediatrics* 123(2) (2009): e274–e281, doi:10.1542/peds. 2008–2251.

38. For a sampling of writing over the past several decades that has explored men's health from a gendered perspective, see Alix Broom and Philip Tovey, *Men's Health: Body, Identity, and Social Context* (The Atrium, Southern Gate, Chichester, West Sussex, UK: Wiley-Blackwell, 2009); W. H. Courtenay, *Dying to Be Men: Psychosocial, Environmental, and Biobehavioral Directions in Promoting the Health of Men and Boys* (New York: Routledge, 2011); Herb Goldberg, *The Hazards of Being Male: Surviving the Myth of Masculine Privilege* (Ojai, CA: Iconoclassics, 2009); William Pollack, *Real Boys: Rescuing Our Sons from the Myths of Boyhood* (New York: Henry Holt, 1999) (see also the initial version of this book published in 1975); Donald Sabo and David F. Gordon, *Men's Health and Illness: Gender, Power, and the Body* (Thousand Oaks, CA: Sage, 1995).

39. Andrea Doucet, *Do Men Mother? Fathering, Care, and Domestic Responsibility* (Toronto: University of Toronto Press, 2006); Brad Harrington, Fred Van Deusen, and Beth Humberd, *The New Dad: Caring, Committed, and Conflicted* (Boston: Boston College Center for Work & Family, 2011); Brad Harrington, Fred Van Deusen, and Jamie Ladge, *The New Dad: Exploring Fatherhood within a Career Context* (Boston: Boston College Center for Work & Family, 2010); Tina Miller, "'It's a Triangle That's Difficult to Square': Men's Intentions and Practices Around Caring, Work, and First-Time Fatherhood," *Fathering* 8, no. 3 (2010): 362–378.

40. Kerstin Aumann, Ellen Galinsky, and Kenneth Matos, *The New Male Mystique* (New York: Families and Work Institute, 2011); see also Beth Humberd, Jamie J. Ladge, and Brad Harrington, "The 'New' Dad: Navigating Fathering Identity Within Organizational Contexts," *Journal of Business and Psychology* 30 (2015): 249–266.

41. Joseph H. Pleck, "Paternal Involvement: Revised Conceptualization and Theoretical Linkages with Child Outcomes," in *The Role of the Father in Child Development*, 5th ed., ed. Michael E. Lamb (New York: Wiley, 2010), 67–107; Joseph H. Pleck and Brian P. Masciadrelli, "Paternal Involvement by U.S. Residential Fathers: Levels, Sources, and Consequences," in *The Role of the Father in Child Development*, 4th ed., ed. Michael E. Lamb (Hoboken, N.J.: Wiley, 2004).

42. Gretchen Livingston, "The Rise of Single Fathers: A Ninefold Increase since 1960," Pew Research Center, July 2, 2013, http://www.pewsocialtrends.org/2013/07/02/the -rise-of-single-fathers/, accessed February 2, 2016; Gretchen Livingston, "Growing Number of Dads Home with the Kids: Biggest Increase Among Those Caring for Family," Pew Research Center, June 5, 2014, http://www.pewsocialtrends.org/2014/06/05/ growing-number-of-dads-home-with-the-kids/, accessed February 2, 2016.

43. Aumann, Galinsky, and Matos, *The New Male Mystique*.

44. Gayle Kaufman, *Superdads: How Fathers Balance Work and Family in the 21st Century* (New York: New York University Press, 2013).

45. Ibid., 7, italics in original.

46. Susan D. Stewart, "Disneyland Dads, Disneyland Moms? How Nonresident Parents Spend Time with Absent Children," *Journal of Family Issues* 20 (1999): 539–556.

47. Jessica Skolnikoff and Robert Engvall, *Youth Athletes, Couch Potatoes, and Helicopter Parents: The Productivity of Play* (Lanham, MD: Rowman & Littlefield, 2014).

48. William Marsiglio and Kevin Roy, *Nurturing Dads: Social Initiatives for Contemporary Fatherhood*, ASA Rose Monograph Series (New York: Russell Sage Foundation, 2012), 66.

49. Michal Al-Yagon, "Fathers' Emotional Resources and Children's Socioemotional and Behavioral Adjustment among Children with Learning Disabilities," *Journal of Child Family Studies* 20 (2011): 569–584; Amanda C. Brody and Leigh Ann Simmons, "Family Resiliency during Childhood Cancer: The Father's Perspective," *Journal of Pediatric Oncology Nursing* 24, no. 3 (2007): 152–165; Juanne N. Clarke, "Father's Home Health Care Work When a Child Has Cancer: I'm Her Dad, I Have to Do It," *Men and Masculinities* 7, no. 4 (2005): 385–404; Karalyn Hill et al., "Fathers' Views and Understanding of Their Roles in Families with a Child with Acute Lymphoblastic Leukaemia: An Interpretative Phenomenological Analysis," *Journal of Health Psychology* 14, no. 8 (2009): 1268–1280; Judith K. Hovey, "The Needs of Fathers Parenting Children with Chronic Conditions," *Journal of Pediatric Oncology Nursing* 20, no. 5 (2003): 245–251; Judith K. Hovey, "Differences in Parenting Needs of Fathers of Children with Chronic Conditions Related to Family Income," *Journal of Child Health Care* 10, no. 1 (2006): 43–54; Ted McNeill, "Fathers of Children with a Chronic Health Condition: Beyond Gender Stereotypes," *Men and Masculinities* 9, no. 4 (2007): 409–424.

50. Clarke, "Father's Home Health Care Work When a Child Has Cancer"; Ann-Christine Hallberg, Anders Beckman, and Anders Håkansson, "Many Fathers Visit the Child Health Care Centre, But Few Take Part in Parents' Groups," *Journal of Child Health Care* 14, no. 3 (2010): 296–303; Hovey, "The Needs of Fathers Parenting Children with Chronic Conditions"; David. J. Sterken, "Uncertainty and Coping in Fathers of Children with Cancer," *Journal of Pediatric Oncology Nursing* 13, no. 2 (1996): 81–88; Linda Beth Tiedje and Cynthia Darling-Fisher, "Promoting Father-Friendly Healthcare," *American Journal of Maternal/Child Nursing* 28 (2003): 350–359; Ware and Raval, "A Qualitative Investigation of Fathers' Experiences of Looking After a Child with a Life-limiting Illness, in Process and Retrospect."

51. Ilana Duvdevany, Eli Buchbinder, and Ilanit Yaacov, "Accepting Disability: The Parenting Experience of Fathers with Spinal Cord Injury (SCI)," *Qualitative Health Research* 18, no. 8 (2008): 1021–1033.

CHAPTER 2   FROM BEING A BOY TO BECOMING A DADDY

1. Richard Louv, *The Last Child in the Woods: Saving Our Children from Nature-Deficit Disorder* (Chapel Hill, NC: Algonquin Books, 2008); Richard Louv, *The Nature Principle: Reconnecting with Life in a Virtual Age* (Chapel Hill, NC: Algonquin Books, 2012).

2. Louise Silvern, Jane Karyl, Lynn Waelde, William F. Hodges, Joanna Starek, Elizabeth Heidt, and Kyung Min, "Retrospective Reports of Parental Partner Abuse: Relationships to Depression, Trauma Symptoms, and Self-esteem among College Students," *Journal of Family Violence 10* (1995): 177–202; see also J. L. Edleson, *Emerging Responses to Children Exposed to Domestic Violence* (Harrisburg, PA: VAWnet, 2006), a project of the National Resource Center on Domestic Violence/Pennsylvania Coalition Against Domestic Violence, http://www.vawnet.org, accessed March 15, 2014.

3. Sherry Hamby, David Finkelhor, Heather Turner, and Richard Ormrod, "Children's Exposure to Intimate Partner Violence and Other Family Violence," *Juvenile Justice Bulletin*, October 2011, U.S. Department of Justice; see also David Finkelhor, Heather Turner, Richard Ormrod, and Sherry L. Hamby, "Violence, Abuse, and Crime Exposure in a National Sample of Children and Youth," *Pediatrics 124 (2009)*: 1411–1423.

4. Katherine M. Kitzmann, Noni K. Gaylord, Aimee R. Holt, and Erin D. Kenny, "Child Witnesses to Domestic Violence: A Meta-analytic Review," *Journal of Consulting and Clinical Psychology* 71 (2003): 339–352.

5. Michael Kimmel, *Guyland: The Inner World of Young Men* (New York: HarperCollins, 2008), 18–27.

6. William Marsiglio, "Making Males Mindful of Their Sexual and Procreative Identities: Using Self-Narratives in Field Settings," *Perspectives on Sexual and Reproductive Health* 35 (2003): 229–233; William Marsiglio and Sally Hutchinson, *Sex, Men, and Babies: Stories of Awareness and Responsibility* (New York: New York University Press, 2002); William Marsiglio and Kevin Roy, *Nurturing Dads: Social Initiatives for Contemporary Fatherhood*, ASA Rose Monograph Series (New York: Russell Sage Foundation, 2012).

7. See Dr. David Bell's op-eds expressing the view that educational and health care organizations are not doing enough to address young men's health care issues, http://www.psmag.com/health-and-behavior/what-are-you-so-afraid-of-men-get-off-the-couch-and-go-to-the-doctor; http://www.psmag.com/health-and-behavior/young-men-and-the-unspoken-danger-of-college-campuses.

8. Cynthia R. Daniels, *The Science and Politics of Male Reproduction* (Oxford: Oxford University Press, 2006).

9. Caitlin Ryan, *Helping Families Support Their Lesbian, Gay, Bisexual, and Transgender (LGBT) Children* (Washington, DC: National Center for Cultural Competence, Georgetown University Center for Child and Human Development, 2009); see also a list of resources at the website *Dads & Kids: Health & Fitness Talk*, http://www.dadsandkidshealth.com/a-dads-guide-to-supporting-lgbt-kids.html, accessed August 28, 2015.

10. See Victorica Hosegood, Linda Richter, and Lynda Clarke, "'. . . I should maintain a healthy life now and not just live as I please . . .': Men's Health and

Fatherhood in Rural South Africa," *American Journal of Men's Health* (2015): 1–12, doi:10.1177/1557988315586440, for a qualitative analysis of how fifty-one Zulu-speaking men in South Africa framed heir experience of becoming fathers relative to approach to their own health.

11. "The World's First Male Pregnancy," https://www.youtube.com/watch?v=AiU -KZ_KADY, accessed February 16, 2016.

12. "First Married Man to Give Birth," Guinness World Records, http://www .guinnessworldrecords.com/world-records/first-married-man-to-give-birth/.

13. "Expecting Fathers Experience Contractions," http://www.youtube.com/watch?v =KHjB8prndf4; "Two Guys Endure Two Hours of Labor Pains," http://www.youtube .com/watch?v=E4h6nphw9B0, accessed February 16, 2016.

14. Lars Plantin, Adepeju Aderemi Olukoya, and Pernilla Ny, "Positive Health Outcomes of Fathers' Involvement in Pregnancy and Childbirth Paternal Support: A Scope Study Literature Review," *Fathering* 9 (2011): 87–102; useful resources for expectant fathers include the American Congress of Obstetricians and Gynecologists' document, http://www.acog.org/Patients/FAQs/A-Fathers-Guide-to-Pregnancy, and the Columbus Obstetricians-Gynecologists Inc., http://www.columbusobgyn.com/patient -education/obstetrics/father's-guide-pregnancy, accessed July 21, 2015.

15. Margareta Widarsson, Gabriella Engsröm, Tanja Tydén, Pranee Lundberg, and Lena Marmstål Hammar, "'Paddling Upstream': Fathers' Involvement during Pregnancy as Described by Expectant Fathers and Mothers," *Journal of Clinical Nursing* 24 (2015): 1059–1068.

16. See the following document prepared by the Royal College of Midwives that targets maternity service staff with the intent of getting fathers more actively involved in maternity care, https://www.rcm.org.uk/sites/default/files/Father%27s%20Guides %20A4_3_0.pdf, accessed July 21, 2015.

17. D. N. Cox, B. K. Wittman, M. Hess, A. G. Ross, J. Lind, and S. Lindahl. 1987. "The Psychological Impact of Diagnostic Ultrasound," *Obstetrics and Gynecology* 70, no. 5 (1987): 673–676; Jan Draper, "'It Was a Real Good Show': The Ultrasound Scan, Fathers, and the Power of Visual Knowledge," *Sociology of Health & Illness* 24 (January 2002): 771–795; Martin P. Johnson and John E. Puddifoot. "Miscarriage: Is Vividness of Visual Imagery a Factor in the Grief Reaction of the Partner?" *British Journal of Health Psychology* 3 (1998): 137–146; Barbara Katz Rothman, *The Tentative Pregnancy: Amniocentesis and the Sexual Politics of Motherhood* (London: Pandora, 1994).

18. M. J. Casper, *The Making of the Unborn Patient: A Social Anatomy of Fetal Surgery* (New Brunswick, NJ: Rutgers University Press, 1998).

19. Janelle S. Taylor, "The Public Foetus and the Family Car: From Abortion Politics to a Volvo Advertisement," *Science as Culture* 3, no. 17 (1993): 601–618; Rosalind Pollack Petchesky, "Foetal Images: The Power of Visual Culture in the Politics of Reproduction," *Feminist Studies* 13, no. 2 (1987): 263–292.

20. Aside from the evolving technologies, the increase in female OBGYNs and ultrasound technicians may alter the way recent cohorts of men experience their prenatal visits.

21. Jacqueline H. Wolf, "Low Breastfeeding Rates and Public Health in the United States," *American Journal of Public Health* 93 (2003): 2000–2010; Julie E. Artis,

"Breastfeed at Your Own Risk," *Contexts* 8 (2009): 28–34; see also American Academy of Pediatrics, "Breastfeeding and the Use of Human Milk," *Pediatrics* 115 (2005): 496–506; see also http://www.babycenter.com/0_how-breastfeeding-benefits-you-and-your-baby_8910.bc, accessed December 12, 2013.

22. Phyllis L. F. Rippeyoung and Mary C. Noonan, "Is Breastfeeding Truly Cost Free? Income Consequences of Breastfeeding for Women," *American Sociological Review* 77 (2012): 244–267; Phyllis L. F. Rippeyoung and Mary C. Noonan, "Breastfeeding and the Gendering of Infant Care," in *Beyond Health, Beyond Choice: Breastfeeding Constraints and Realities*, ed. B. L. Hausman, P. Hall Smith, and M. Labbok (New Brunswick, NJ: Rutgers University Press, 2012).

23. Pamela L. Jordan and Virginia R. Wall, "Breastfeeding and Fathers: Illuminating the Darker Side," *Birth* 17 (1990): 210–213.

24. Rippeyoung and Noonan, "Breastfeeding and the Gendering of Infant Care."

25. Ibid.

26. Rippeyoung and Noonan, "Is Breastfeeding Truly Cost Free?"; Rippeyoung and Noonan, "Breastfeeding and the Gendering of Infant Care."

27. Joan B. Wolf, "Is Breast Really Best? Risk and Total Motherhood in the National Breastfeeding Awareness Campaign," *Journal of Health Politics, Policy, and Law* 32 (2007): 596–636.

28. Brigitte Jordan, "Authoritative Knowledge and Its Construction," in *Childbirth and Authoritative Knowledge: Cross-Cultural Perspectives*, ed. Robbie E. David-Floyd and Carolyn F. Sargent (Berkeley: University of California Press, 1997), 55–79.

29. Judith Walzer Leavitt, *Make Room for Daddy: The Journey from Waiting Room to Birthing Room* (Chapel Hill: University of North Carolina Press, 2009).

CHAPTER 3   ROUTINES, RITUALS, AND CARE

1. See Pawlak Roman, Ding Qin, and Sovyanhadi Marta, "Pregnancy Outcome and Breastfeeding Pattern among Vegans, Vegetarians, and Non-vegetarians," *Eliven: Journal of Dietetics Research and Nutrition* 1 (2014): 1–4. Although Jeremy was uncertain about whether he had prebirth discussions with his wife about breast-feeding, such discussions can be connected to a mother's dietary habits. Children born to vegan and vegetarian mothers are more likely to be breast-fed than children born to mothers who eat meat (93.3 and 89.1 percent to 74.4 percent, respectively). Because women on non-meat diets are susceptible to having vitamin B12 and iron deficiencies, which can put their child at risk for low birth weight, fathers can contribute to their child's health by encouraging their partners to consult health and nutrition specialists to make sure they supplement their diets appropriately.

2. Richard Louv, *The Last Child in the Woods: Saving Our Children from Nature-Deficit Disorder* (Chapel Hill, NC: Algonquin Books, 2008); Richard Louv, *The Nature Principle: Reconnecting with Life in a Virtual Age* (Chapel Hill, NC: Algonquin Books, 2012).

3. Molly Watson, "What's a Locavore," About Food, http://localfoods.about.com/od/localfoodsglossary/g/locavore.htm, accessed November 29, 2013.

4. William Marsiglio and Kevin Roy, *Nurturing Dads: Social Initiatives for Contemporary Fatherhood*. ASA Rose Monograph Series (New York: Russell Sage Foundation, 2012).

5. M. Gillman, "Family Dinner and Diet Quality among Older Children and Adolescents," *Archives of Family Medicine* 9 (2000): 235–240.

6. See news article highlighting the trend of fathers getting their children more involved in sharing cooking duties with them: Debra Samuels, "Food-savvy Dads at the Stove," *Boston Globe*, June 16, 2015, https://www.bostonglobe.com/lifestyle/food -dining/2015/06/16/food-savvy-dads-stove/0aW6i0XDQOS71ByZI0xMEM/story .html, retrieved June 17, 2015.

7. http://www.merriam-webster.com/dictionary/foodways.

8. Linda Keller Brown and Kay Mussell, "Introduction," in *Ethnic and Regional Foodways in the United States: The Performance of Group Identity*, ed. Linda Keller Brown and Kay Mussell (Knoxville: University of Tennessee Press), 3–15.

9. Zilkia Janer, *Latino Food Culture* (Westport, CT: Greenwood, 2008).

10. Ibid.

11. Jonathan Deutsch and Rachel D. Saks, *Jewish American Food Culture* (Westport, CT: Greenwood, 2008), 123.

12. Ibid.

13. Ibid.

14. See also the National Obesity Observatory report on ethnic variations in obesity for the population in the United Kingdom, http://www.noo.org.uk/uploads/doc/vid _9444_Obesity_and_ethnicity_270111.pdf, accessed November 29, 2013.

15. United States Department of Agriculture, Nutrition Evidence Library, http://www .nel.gov/evidence.cfm?evidence_summary_id=250379, accessed November 29, 2013; Serena Tonstad, Terry Butler, Ru Yan, and Gary E. Fraser, "Type of Vegetarian Diet, Body Weight, and Prevalence of Type 2 Diabetes," *Diabetes Care* 32 (2009): 791–796.

16. Molly Watson, "Community-Supported Agriculture (CSA)," About Food, http:// localfoods.about.com/od/localfoodsglossary/g/csa_glossary.htm, accessed November 29, 2013.

17. Sabrina L. Gustafson and Ryan E. Rhodes, "Parental Correlates of Physical Activity in Children and Early Adolescents," *Sports Medicine* 36 (2006): 79–97.

18. Josephine Fraser, Helen Skouteris, Marita McCabe, Lina A. Ricciardelli, Jeannette Milgrom, and Louise Baur, "Paternal Influences on Children's Weight Gain: A Systematic Review," *Fathering* 9 (2011): 252–267; R. Stein, L. Epstein, H. Raynor, C. Kilanowski, and R. Paluch, "The Influence of Parenting Change on Pediatric Weight Control," *Obesity* 13 (2005): 1749–1755; Milissa Wake, Jan M. Nicholson, Pollyanna Hardy, and Katherine Smith, "Preschooler Obesity and Parenting Styles of Mothers and Fathers: Australian National Population Study," *Pediatrics* 120, no. 6 (2007): e1520–e1527.

19. Jay Coakley, "The Good Father: Parental Expectations and Youth Sports," *Leisure Studies* 25 (2006): 153–163, 159; see also Michael Messner, *It's All for the Kids: Gender, Family, and Youth Sports* (Berkeley: University of California Press, 2009).

20. Donald Sabo and Phil Veliz, *Go Out and Play: Youth Sports in America* (East Meadow, NY: Women's Sports Foundation, 2008); see also Messner, *It's All for the Kids.*

21. Sabo and Veliz, *Go Out and Play*; see also http://www.womenssportsfoundation
.org/sitecore/content/home/research/articles-and-reports/mental-and-physical
-health/go-out-and-play.aspx, accessed July 8, 2015.

22. Bruce Kelley and Carl Carchia, "Hey, Data Data—Swing!" ESPN, July 16, 2013,
http://espn.go.com/espn/story/_/id/9469252/hidden-demographics-youth-sports
-espn-magazine, accessed February 5, 2016.

23. Lucas Gottzén and Tamar Kremer-Sadlik, "Fatherhood and Youth Sports: A Balancing Act between Care and Expectations," *Gender & Society* 26 (2012): 639–664.

24. Jessica Skolnikoff and Robert Engvall, *Youth Athletes, Couch Potatoes, and Helicopter
Parents: The Productivity of Play* (Lanham, MD: Rowman & Littlefield, 2014).

25. William Marsiglio, *Men on a Mission: Valuing Youth Work in Our Communities* (Baltimore: Johns Hopkins University Press, 2008); see also the Centers for Disease Control and Prevention's website, which provides information about safety issues for youth,
http://www.cdc.gov/family/kids/, accessed May 16, 2014.

26. Kansas Department of Health and Environment, SafeKids, http://www.kdheks
.gov/news/web_archives/2012/01232012.htm, accessed May 31, 2013.

27. Eric J. Crossen, Brenna Lewis, and Benjamin D. Hoffman, "Preventing Gun Injuries in Children," *Pediatrics in Review* 36 (2015): 43–51.

28. "My First Rifle," *Daily Mail*, April 30, 2013, http://www.dailymail.co.uk/news/
article-2317512/Kentucky-boy-5-shoots-sister-Caroline-Starks-2-child-size-22-caliber
-rifle-given-GIFT.html, accessed May 31, 2013.

29. Gallup Topics, Guns, http://www.gallup.com/poll/1645/guns.aspx, accessed
May 20, 2015.

30. Lydia Saad, "Self-Reported Gun Ownership in U.S. Is Highest Since 1993," Gallup
Topics, Politics, http://www.gallup.com/poll/150353/self-reported-gun-ownership
-highest-1993.aspx, accessed May 31, 2013.

31. Centers for Disease Control and Prevention, Injury Prevention & Control: Motor
Vehicle Safety, http://www.cdc.gov/motorvehiclesafety/teen_drivers/teendrivers
_factsheet.html, accessed February 6, 2016.

32. National Capital Poison Center, Poison Statistics, http://www.poison.org/stats/,
accessed May 20, 2015.

33. Andrea Doucet, *Do Men Mother? Fathering, Care, and Domestic Responsibility*
(Toronto: University of Toronto Press, 2006).

34. Lisa L. Olsen et al. "Fathers' Views on Their Financial Situations, Father-Child Activities, and Preventing Child Injuries," *American Journal of Men's Health* 9 (2015): 15–25.

35. Takeo Fujiwara, Makiko Okuyama, and Kunihiko Takahashi, "Paternal Involvement in Childcare and Unintentional Injury of Young Children: A Population-based
Cohort Study in Japan," *International Journal of Epidemiology* 39 (2010): 588–597. For
an extensive discussion of the potential links between fathers' involvement and childhood injuries see, Lenna Nepomnyaschy and Louis Donnelly, "Father Involvement and
Childhood Injuries," *Journal of Marriage and Family* 77 (2015): 628–646.

36. David C. Schwebel and Carl M. Brezausek, "How Do Mothers and Fathers Influence Pediatric Injury Risk in Middle Childhood?" *Journal of Pediatric Psychology* 35
(2010): 806–813.

37. William Marsiglio, Kevin Roy, and Greer Litton Fox, "Conceptualizing Situated Fatherhood: A Spatially-Sensitive and Social Approach," in *Situated Fathering: A Focus on Physical and Social Spaces*, edited by William Marsiglio, Kevin Roy, and Greer Litton Fox (Lanham, MD: Rowman & Littlefield, 2005), 3–26.

38. American College of Sports Medicine, "Actively Moving America to Better Health," 2015, http://americanfitnessindex.org/wp-content/uploads/2015/05/acsm _afireport_2015.pdf, accessed February 7, 2016.

39. Ibid., 7.

40. For the full ranking see American College of Sports Medicine, 2015, 8. Some select rankings follow: (1) Washington–Arlington–Alexandria, DC–VA–MD–WV; (2) Minneapolis–St. Paul–Bloomington, MN–WI; (3) San Diego–Carlsbad, CA; (14) Atlanta–Sandy Springs–Roswell, GA; (23) Los Angeles–Long Beach–Anaheim, CA; (36) Orlando–Kissimmee–Sanford, FL; (48) Oklahoma City, OK; (49) Memphis, TN–MS–AR; (50) Indianapolis–Carmel–Anderson, IN.

CHAPTER 4   TAKING STOCK AND ACHIEVING PERSONAL GROWTH

1. Jeffrey Sobal, "Men, Meat, and Marriage: Models of Masculinity," *Food and Foodways* 13 (2005): 135–158. http://www.vrg.org/.

2. Frank Newport, "In U.S., 5% Consider Themselves Vegetarians," Gallup Topics, Well-Being, July 26, 2012, http://www.gallup.com/poll/156215/consider-themselves -vegetarians.aspx, accessed July 4, 2013.

3. Richard Rogers, "Beasts, Burgers, and Hummers: Meat and the Crisis of Masculinity in Contemporary Television Advertisements," *Environmental Communication* 2 (2008): 281–301.

4. Zachary A. Kramer, "Of Meat and Manhood," *Washington University Law Review* 89 (2011): 287–322.

5. http://www.youtube.com/watch?v=A4zmGohh1oQ, accessed December 13, 2013.

6. This show evolved into *Man v. Food Nation*, http://www.travelchannel.com/shows/ man-v-food/episodes, accessed February 8, 2016.

7. Mari Kate Mycek, "Man v. Food: Representations of Meat and Masculinity," *Feminist Wire*, April 18, 2012, http://thefeministwire.com/2012/04/man-v-food-representations -of-meat-and-masculinity/, accessed July 8, 2013.

8. Paul Rozin, Julia M. Hormes, Myles S. Faith, and Brian Wansink, "Is Meat Male? A Quantitative Multi-Method Framework to Establish Metaphoric Relationships," *Journal of Consumer Research* 39 (2012): 629–643.

9. Ahmed Jamal, Israel T. Agaku, Erin O'Conner, Brian A. King, John B. Kenemer, and Linda Neff, "Current Cigarette Smoking among Adults—United States, 2005–2013," Centers for Disease Control and Prevention, *Morbidity and Mortality Weekly Report* 63, no.47 (2014).

10. Mike Vuolo and Jeremy Staff, "Parent and Child Cigarette Use: A Longitudinal Multigenerational Study," *Pediatrics* 132 (2013): 1–10. Jo Leonardi-Bee, John Britton, and Andrea Venn, "Secondhand Smoke and Adverse Fetal Outcomes in Nonsmoking

Pregnant Women: A Meta Analysis," *Pediatrics* 127, no. 4 (2011): 734–741; Mahideyeh Mojibyan, Mehran Karimi, Reza Bidaki, and Asghar Zare, "Exposure to Second-Hand Smoke during Pregnancy and Preterm Delivery," *International Journal of High Risk Behaviors and Addiction* 1. no. 4 (2013): 149–153. Shama Khan, Ahmed A. Arif, Jamie N. Laditka, and Elizabeth F. Racine, "Prenatal Exposure to Secondhand Smoke May Increase the Risk of Postpartum Depressive Symptoms," *Journal of Public Health* (2015), doi:10.1093/pubmed/fdv083.

11. TaraCulp-Ressler, "Former 'Marlboro Man' Who Helped Sell Cigarettes in the 1970s Dies From Smoking-Related Disease," *Think Progress*, January 27, 2014, http://thinkprogress.org/health/2014/01/27/3207091/marlboro-man-dies-smoking/, accessed September 15, 2015.

12. Robert Klara, "The Marlboro Man Still Sells Cigarettes: E-cigarettes Get Tough," April 11, 2013, *Adweek*, http://www.adweek.com/news/advertising-branding/marlboro-man-still-sells-cigarettes-148416, accessed February 8, 2016.

13. *Morbidity and Mortality Weekly Report*, "Percentage of Persons Aged >= 18 Years Who Were Current Cigarette Smokers,* by Selected Characteristics—National Health Interview Survey, United States, 2005 and 2010," http://www.cdc.gov/mmwr/pdf/wk/mm6035.pdf#page=21, accessed August 15, 2013.

14. William. I. Thomas and Dorothy Swain Thomas, *The Child in America: Behavior Problems and Programs* (New York: Knopf, 1928).

15. A full-distance triathlon consists of swimming 2.4 miles (3.8 km), biking 112 miles (180.2 km), and running 26.2 miles (42.2 km) in immediate succession. The term IRON-MAN is a corporate brand name that is trademarked by World Triathlon Corporation (WTC).

16. U.S. Department of Veterans Affairs, 2015, http://www.ptsd.va.gov/professional/provider-type/doctors/screening-and-referral.asp. The main reasons VA patients refuse mental health care include: "discomfort with the idea of seeing a psychologist or psychiatrist, a perceived stigma associated with treatment, previous negative experiences with mental health providers, negative attitudes towards health care agencies, a lack of confidence in the helpfulness of counseling, or a reluctance to open up old emotional wounds."

17. Drug Policy Alliance, "Healing a Broken System: Veterans Battling Addiction and Incarceration," Issue Brief, November 4, 2009; Andrew Golub, Peter Vazan, Alexander S. Bennett, and Hilary J. Liberty, "Unmet Need for Treatment of Substance Use Disorders and Serious Psychological Distress among Veterans: A Nationwide Analysis Using the NSDUH," *Military Medicine* 178 (2013): 107–114; Steven L. Sayers, "Family Reintegration Difficulties and Couples Therapy for Military Veterans and Their Spouses," *Cognitive and Behavioral Practice* 18 (2011): 108–119; Joshua E. Wilk, Paul D. Bliese, Paul Y. Kim, Jeffrey L. Thomas, Dennis McGurk, and Charles W. Hoge, "Relationship of Combat Experiences to Alcohol Misuse among U.S. Soldiers Returning from the Iraq War," *Drug and Alcohol Dependence* 108 (2009): 115–121.

18. Office of the Deputy Under Secretary of Defense, 2011 Demographics: Profile of the Military Community, Updated November 2012, http://www.militaryonesource.mil/12038/MOS/Reports/2011_Demographics_Report.pdf, accessed August 23, 2013.

19. Christal Presley, *Thirty Days with My Father: Finding Peace from Wartime PTSD* (Deerfield Beach, FL: Health Communications, 2012). See also Moni Basu, "A Daughter Faces Demons of Father's War," November 4, 2012, CNN, http://www.cnn.com/2012/11/04/us/veteran-daughter-ptsd/, accessed February 8, 2016.

20. Lauren E. Glaze, and Laura M. Maruschak, "Parents in Prison and Their Minor Children," Bureau of Justice Statistics Special Report, revised March 30, 2010, http://www.bjs.gov/content/pub/pdf/pptmc.pdf, accessed September 25, 2015.

21. W. H. Courtenay, "Constructions of Masculinity and Their Influence on Men's Well-being: A Theory of Gender and Health," *Social Science and Medicine* 50 (2000): 1385–1401; see also Ronald. F. Levant, David. J. Wimer, Christine M. Williams, K. Bryant Smalley, and Delilah Noronha, "The Relationships between Masculinity Variables, Health Risk Behaviors and Attitudes Toward Seeking Psychological Help," *International Journal of Men's Health* 8 (2009): 3–21.

22. Courtenay, "Constructions of Masculinity and Their Influence on Men's Well-being."

23. Michael Messner, "The Life of a Man's Seasons: Male Identity in the Life Course of the Athlete," in *Changing Men: New Directions in Research on Men and Masculinity,* ed. Michael S. Kimmel (Thousand Oaks, CA: Sage, 1987), 54–67.

24. Michael Messner, "Masculinities and Athletic Careers," *Gender & Society* 3 (1989): 71–88.

25. Emily Senay and Rob Waters, *From Boys to Men: A Women's Guide to the Health of Husbands, Partners, Sons, Fathers, and Brothers* (New York: Scribner, 2004).

26. Kevin C. Davis, W. Douglas Evans, and Kian Kamyab, "Effectiveness of a National Campaign to Promote Parent-child Communication about Sex," *Health Education & Behavior* 40 (2013): 97–106.

27. Alzheimer's Society, "What Is Dementia?" http://www.alzheimers.org.uk/site/scripts/documents_info.php?documentID=106, accessed July 8, 2013.

28. Lenard I. Lesser, Deborah A. Cohen, and Robert H. Brook, "Changing Eating Habits for the Medical Profession," *JAMA* 308 (2012): 983–984.

29. Samantha K. Brooks, Clare Gerada, and Trudie Chalder, "Review of Literature on the Mental Health of Doctors: Are Specialist Services Needed?" *Journal of Mental Health* 20 (2011): 146–156; Erica Frank, Holly Biola, and Carol A. Burnett, "Mortality Rates and Causes among U.S. Physicians," *American Journal of Preventive Medicine* 19 (2000): 155–159.

30. Lisa J. Merlo and Mark S. Gold. 2008. "Prescription Opioid Abuse and Dependence among Physicians: Hypotheses and Treatment," *Harvard Review of Psychiatry* 16 (2008): 181–194.

31. Frank, Biola, and Burnett, "Mortality Rates and Causes among U.S. Physicians."

32. Ibid., 158.

33. U. A. Ajani, P. A. Lutofuo, J. M. Gaziano, I. M. Lee, A. Spelsberg, J. E. Buring, W. C. Willett, and J. E. Manson, 2004, "Body Mass Index and Mortality among US Male Physicians," *Annals of Epidemiology* 14 (2004): 731–739.

34. Mohsen Bazargan, Marian Makar, Shahrzad Bazargan-Hejazi, Chizobam Ani, and Kenneth E. Wolf, "Preventive, Lifestyle, and Personal Health Behaviors among Physicians," *Academic Psychiatry* 33 (2009): 289–295.

35. Erik H. Erikson, *Life History and the Historical Moment* (New York: Norton, 1975).

36. William Marsiglio, *Men on a Mission: Valuing Youth Work in Our Communities* (Baltimore: Johns Hopkins University Press, 2008), 93; see also Ed de St. Aubin, Dan P. McAdams, and Kim Tae-Chang, *The Generative Society: Caring for Future Generations* (Washington, DC: American Psychological Association, 2004).

CHAPTER 5   CHRONIC CHALLENGES

1. Americans with Disabilities Act of 1990, as amended, http://www.ada.gov/pubs/adastatute08.htm.

2. Coleen A. Boyle, Sheree Boulet, Laura A. Schieve, Robin A. Cohen, Stephen J. Blumberg, Marshalyn, Yeargin-Allsopp, Susanna, Visser, and Michael D. Kogan, "Trends in the Prevalence of Developmental Disabilities in US Children, 1997–2008," *Pediatrics* 127 (2011): 1034–1042. The National Health Interview Surveys draw on self-reported data from a "knowledge adult family member" to determine whether any of the conditions apply to a randomly selected child age three to seventeen living in the household: attention deficit hyperactivity disorder, intellectual disability, cerebral palsy, autism, seizures, stuttering or stammering, moderate to profound hearing loss, blindness, learning disorders, and/or other developmental delays.

3. Child Trends, "Autism Spectrum Disorders," 2013, http://www.childtrends.org/?indicators=autism-spectrum-disorders, accessed February 9, 2016.

4. S. Visser, M. Danielson, R. H. Bitsko, J. R. Kogan, M. D., R. M. Ghandour, R. Perou, and S. J. Blumberg, "Trends in the Parent-Report of Health Care Provider-Diagnosis and Medication Treatment for ADHD disorder: United States, 2003–2011," *Journal of the American Academy of Child and Adolescent Psychiatry* 53, no.1 (2014): 34–46.e2; for more information see http://www.cdc.gov/ncbddd/adhd/features/key-findings-adhd72013.html.

5. Samuele Cortese, Maria Olazagasti, Rachel Klein, F. Castellanos, Ericka Proal, and Salvatore Mannuzza, "Obesity in Men with Childhood ADHD: A 33-Year Controlled, Prospective, Follow-up Study," *Pediatrics* 131 (2013): 1731–1738.

6. Elaine E. MacDonald and Richard P. Hastings, "Fathers of Children with Developmental Disabilities," in *The Role of the Father in Child Development*, 5th ed., ed. Michael E. Lamb (Hoboken, NJ: Wiley, 2010), 486–516.

7. Elaine Bass Jenks, "Explaining Disability: Parents' Stories of Raising Children with Visual Impairments in a Sighted World," *Journal of Contemporary Ethnography* 34 (2005): 143–169.

8. Majella Kilkey and Harriet Clarke, "Disabled Men and Fathering: Opportunities and Constraints," *Community, Work & Family* 13 (2010): 127–146; see also Aaron Bonsall, "Fathering Occupations: An Analysis of Narrative Accounts of Fathering Children with Special Needs," *Journal of Occupational Science* 21, no. 4 (2014): 504–518.

9. William Marsiglio and Kevin Roy, *Nurturing Dads: Social Initiatives for Contemporary Fatherhood*, ASA Rose Monograph Series (New York: Russell Sage Foundation, 2012).

10. NHS, "Treating Cystic Fibrosis," http://www.nhs.uk/Conditions/cystic-fibrosis/Pages/Treatment.aspx, accessed February 16, 2016.

11. Robert M. Veatch, "Models for Ethical Medicine in a Revolutionary Age," *Hastings Center Report* 2 (1972): 5–7.

12. Bonsall, "Fathering Occupations."

13. Erik Ortiz, "An Amazing Moment," *New York Daily News*, March 31, 2013, http://www.nydailynews.com/life-style/health/ore-teen-syndrome-scales-mount-everest-article-1.1303959, accessed August 6, 2013.

CHAPTER 6   COPARENTING

1. Mark E. Feinberg, "The Internal Structure and Ecological Context of Coparenting: A Framework for Research and Intervention," *Parenting: Science and Practice* 3 (2003): 95–131, quote on page 96.

2. William Marsiglio and Kevin Roy, *Nurturing Dads: Social Initiatives for Contemporary Fatherhood*, ASA Rose Monograph Series (New York: Russell Sage Foundation, 2012), 21.

3. Mark E. Feinberg, "Coparenting and the Transition to Parenthood: A Framework for Prevention," *Clinical Child and Family Psychology Review* 5 (2002): 173–195.

4. Joseph H. Pleck, "Paternal Involvement: Revised Conceptualization and Theoretical Linkages with Child Outcomes," in *The Role of the Father in Child Development*, 5th ed., ed. Michael E. Lamb (New York: Wiley, 2010), 67–107.

5. Gayle Kaufman, *Superdads: How Fathers Balance Work and Family in the 21st Century* (New York: New York University Press, 2013); Marsiglio and Roy, *Nurturing Dads*; Jeremy A. Smith, *The Daddy Shift: How Stay-at-Home-Dads, Breadwinning Moms, and Shared Parenting Are Transforming the American Family* (Boston: Beacon, 2009).

6. Hannah Seligson, "Don't Call Him Mom, or an Imbecile," *New York Times*, February 23, 2012, http://www.nytimes.com/2013/02/24/business/fathers-seek-advertising-that-does-not-ridicule.html?pagewanted=all&_r=0, accessed March 17, 2014.

7. Michael Kimmel, *Guyland: The Inner World of Young Men* (New York: HarperCollins, 2008), 18–27.

8. Sarah M. Allen and Alan J. Hawkins, "Maternal Gatekeeping: Mothers' Beliefs and Behaviors That Inhibit Greater Father Involvement in Family Work," *Journal of Marriage and Family* 6, no. 1 (1999): 199–212; Jay Fagan and Marina Barnett, "The Relationship between Maternal Gatekeeping, Paternal Competence, Mothers' Attitudes about the Father Role, and Father Involvement," *Journal of Family Issues* 24 (2003):1020–1043; Sarah J. Schoppe-Sullivan, Geoffrey L. Brown, Elizabeth A. Cannon, Sarah C. Mangelsdorf, and Margaret Szewczyk Sokolowski, "Maternal Gatekeeping, Coparenting Quality, and Fathering Behavior in Families with Infants," *Journal of Family Psychology* 22 (2008): 389–398; Bharathi Zvara, Sarah J. Schoppe-Sullivan, and Claire Kamp Dush, "Fathers' Involvement in Child Health Care: Associations with Prenatal Involvement, Parents' Beliefs, and Maternal Gatekeeping," *Family Relations* 62 (2013): 649–661.

9. William Marsiglio, *Stepdads: Stories of Hope, Love, and Repair* (Lanham, MD: Rowman & Littlefield, 2004).

10. Alexis J. Walker and Lori A. McGraw, "Who is Responsible for Responsible Fathering?" *Journal of Marriage and Family* 62 (2000): 563–570.

11. William L. Coleman, Craig Garfield, and American Academy of Pediatrics, Committee on Psychosocial Aspects of Child and Family Health, "Fathers and Pediatricians: Enhancing Men's Roles in the Care and Development of Their Children," *Pediatrics* 113, no. 5 (2004): 1406–1411.

12. "Household Data Annual Averages, 11. Employed Persons by Detailed Occupation, Sex, Race, and Hispanic or Latino Ethnicity," http://www.bls.gov/cps/cpsaat11.pdf, accessed February 12, 2016.

13. See Barbara Barzansky and Sylvia I. Etzel, "Medical Schools in the United States, 2013–2014," *JAMA* 312(22) (2004): 2419–2426; https://www.aamc.org/download/321536/data/factstable29.pdf, accessed May 30, 2015.

14. American Academy of Pediatrics, "Additional Characteristics of Pediatricians: Comparisons Across Time, II. Personal Characteristics of Pediatricians," https://www.aap.org/en-us/professional-resources/Research/Pages/PS43_Additional_Characteristics_of_Pediatricians.aspx, accessed February 12, 2016.

15. U.S. Bureau of Labor Statistics, "Women in the Labor Force: A Databook," February 2013, http://www.bls.gov/cps/wlf-databook-2012.pdf, accessed September 9, 2013.

16. http://www.bls.gov/cps/cpsaat11.pdf, accessed May 30, 2015.

17. Robert. W. Ortiz, Tim Green, and Hee-Jeong Lim, "Families and Home Computer Use: Exploring Parent Perceptions of the Importance of Current Technology," *Urban Education,* 46, no. 2 (2011): 202–215; Rong Wang, Suzanne M. Bianchi, and Sara B. Raley, "Teenagers' Internet Use and Family Rules: A Research Note," *Journal of Marriage and Family* 67 (2005): 1249–1258.

18. Ortiz, Green, and Lim, "Families and Home Computer Use."

19. Interagency Youth Working Group, *Mobile Technology for Health*, Youth Lens on Reproductive Health and HIV/AIDS, no. 38 (Research Triangle Park, NC, 2013)

20. Edward A. Witt, Adam J. Massman, and Linda A. Jackson, "Trends in Youth's Video-game Playing, Overall Computer Use, and Communication Technology Use: The Impact of Self-Esteem and the Big Five Personality Factors," *Computers in Human Behavior* 27 (2011): 763–769; see also "Home Computer Access and Internet Use," Child Trends Data Bank, http://www.childtrends.org/?indicators=home-computer-access&utm_source=E-News%3A+Family+Meals+Are+All+They%27re+Cracked+Up+to+Be&utm_campaign=E-News+9+19+13&utm_medium=email, accessed September 19, 2013.

21. Mary Madden, Amanda Lenhart, Maeve Duggan, Sandra Cortesi, and Urs Gasser, "Teens and Technology," Pew Research Center, 2013, http://www.pewinternet.org/Reports/2013/Teens-and-Tech.aspx, accessed September 2, 2013.

22. Lisa Hartling, Andrea Milne, Lisa Tjosvold, Dawn Wrightson, Jennifer Gallivan, and Amand S. Newton, "A Systematic Review of Interventions to Support Siblings of Children with Chronic Illness or Disability," *Journal of Pediatrics and Child Health* (2010), doi:10.1111/j.1440–1754.2010.01771.x.

23. "The Vaccine War," *Frontline*, PBS, April 27, 2010, http://www.pbs.org/wgbh/pages/frontline/vaccines/, accessed September 27, 2013.

24. "Dr. Carson, Dr. Paul, and 'Dr.' Trump on Vaccines," September 17, 2015, http://www.wsj.com/video/dr-carson-dr-paul-and-dr-trump-on-vaccines/6FA5E538-4F96-44CC-A568-2E1B709D2927.html; Mara Liasson, "5 Things the Vaccine Debacle Reveals About the 2016 Presidential Field," NPR, February 5, 2015, http://www.npr.org/sections/itsallpolitics/2015/02/05/383904342/5-things-the-vaccine-debacle-reveal-about-the-2016-presidential-field, accessed February 12, 2016.

25. "2015 Sexually Transmitted Diseases Treatment Guidelines," Centers for Disease Control and Prevention, http://www.cdc.gov/std/tg2015/hpv.htm, accessed September 2, 2015; see also Amy Norton, "Parents' Worries About HPV Vaccine on the Rise: Study," March 18, 2013, http://consumer.healthday.com/mental-health-information-25/behavior-health-news-56/parents-worries-about-hpv-vaccine-on-the-rise-study-674474.html, accessed February 12, 2016; and the Henry J. Kaiser Family Foundation, "The HPV Vaccine: Access and Use in the U.S.," September 3, 2015, http://kff.org/womens-health-policy/fact-sheet/the-hpv-vaccine-access-and-use-in/, accessed February 12, 2016.

CHAPTER 7   MAKING PROACTIVE DADS

1. Bruce Barcott, "Senseless," *Bicycling*, June 2013, http://www.bicycling.com/sites/default/files/uploads/BI-June-13-Helmet.pdf, accessed February 12, 2016.

2. William Marsiglio, *Men on a Mission: Valuing Youth Work in Our Communities* (Baltimore: Johns Hopkins University Press, 2008); William Marsiglio and Kevin Roy, *Nurturing Dads: Social Initiatives for Contemporary Fatherhood*, ASA Rose Monograph Series (New York: Russell Sage Foundation, 2012); William Marsiglio, Kevin Roy, and Greer Litton Fox, "Conceptualizing Situated Fatherhood: A Spatially Sensitive and Social Approach," in *Situated Fathering: A Focus on Physical and Social Spaces*, ed. William Marsiglio, Kevin Roy, and Greer Litton Fox (Lanham, MD: Rowman & Littlefield, 2005), 3–26.

3. MADD, "Rebecca (Beckie) Brown, 1940–2012," http://www.madd.org/about-us/history/rebecca-beckie-brown.html.

4. MADD, MADD Milestones, http://www.madd.org/about-us/history/madd-milestones.pdf, accessed September 23, 2013.

5. A few years ago, three dads in Connecticut had a series of productive conversations about childhood obesity and the excess sugary drinks children consume. It led the trio to invent an alternative to soda and sports drinks. The protein-infused water product is called Trimino and hit the shelves in February 2014. See http://foxct.com/2015/06/16/three-dads-say-theyve-created-a-refreshing-change-for-young-athletes/, accessed June 17, 2015.

6. https://www.facebook.com/The-Boys-Initiative-181402825206162/info/?tab=page_info, accessed February 16, 2016.

7. Marsiglio, *Men on a Mission*; Marsiglio and Roy, *Nurturing Dads*.

8. Diana T. Cohen, *Iron Dads: Managing Work, Family, and Endurance Sport Identities* (New Brunswick, NJ: Rutgers University Press, 2016).

9. Craig F. Garfield, "Fathers and the Well-Child Visit," *Pediatrics* 117 (2006): 637–645.

10. Pew Center on the States, "States and the New Federal Home Visiting Initiative: An Assessment from the Starting Line," August, 2011, http://www.pewtrusts .org/~/media/legacy/uploadedfiles/wwwpewtrustsorg/reports/home_visiting/ homevisitingaugust2011reportpdf.pdf/. Among these states, at least thirty-four reported investing in at least two prenatal and early childhood home visiting programs. Twenty-one states funded three or more programs.

11. Children's Trust Strengthening Families 2015 Annual Report. http://childrenstrust ma.org/uploads/files/2015_Annual_ReportV3-webfinal.pdf, accessed February 14, 2016.

12. Katherine L. Wisner., Dorothy K. Y. Sit, Mary C. McShea, David M. Rizzo, Rebecca A. Zoretich, Carolyn L. Hughes, Heather F. Eng, James F. Luther, Stephen R. Wisniewski, Michelle L. Costantino, Andrea L. Confer, Eydie L. Moses-Kolko, Christopher S. Famy, and Barbara H. Hanusa, "Onset Timing, Thoughts of Self-harm, and Diagnoses in Postpartum Women With Screen-Positive Depression Findings," *JAMA Psychiatry* 70, no. 5 (2013): 490–498, doi:10.1001/jamapsychiatry.2013.87; see also http:// www.npr.org/blogs/health/2013/03/13/174214166/postpartum-depression-affects-1-in -7-women; http://www.apa.org/pi/women/programs/depression/postpartum.aspx.

13. James F. Paulson, and Sharnail D. Bazemore, "Prenatal and Postpartum Depression in Fathers and Its Association with Maternal Depression: A Meta-analysis," *JAMA* 303 (2010): 1961–1969; Karen-leigh Edward, David Castle, Cally Mills, Leigh Davis, and June Casey, "An Integrative Review of Paternal Depression," *American Journal of Men's Health* 9 (2015): 26–34; see also http://www.postpartummen.com/we-men-do.htm, accessed February 24, 2016.

14. Paulson and Bazemore, "Prenatal and Postpartum Depression in Fathers and Its Association with Maternal Depression"; Edward, Castle, Mills, Davis, and Casey, "An Integrative Review of Paternal Depression."

15. Paul Ramchandani, Alan Stein, Thomas G. O'Conner, and the ALSPAC study team, "Paternal Depression in the Postnatal Period and Child Development: A Prospective Population Study," *Lancet* 365 (2015): 2201–2205.

16. David L. Hill, *Dad to Dad: Parenting Like a Pro: Expert Advice, Guidance, and Insight from a Pediatrician-Dad* (Elk Grove, IL: American Academy of Pediatrics, 2012).

17. Linda Beth Tiedje and Cynthia Darling-Fisher, "Promoting Father-friendly Healthcare," *Maternal/Child Nursing* 28 (2003): 350–359.

18. See Texas Department of State Health Services, https://www.dshs.state.tx.us/ wichd/tng/desc-gen.shtm and http://www.dadsandkidshealth.com/uploads/3/0/3/ 1/30319129/father_friendliness.pdf, accessed September 3, 2015.

19. Jennifer H. Elder, Susan O. Donaldson, John Kairalla, Gregory Valcante, Roxanna Bendixen, Richard Ferdig, Erica Self, Jeffrey Walker, Christina Palau, and Michele Serrano, "In-home Training for Fathers of Children with Autism: A Follow Up Study and Evaluation of Four Individual Training Components," *Journal of Child and Family Studies* 20 (2011): 263–271; Jennifer. H. Elder, Gregory Valcante, Hassein Yarandi, Deborah

White, and Timothy H. Elder, "Evaluating In-home Training for Fathers of Children with Autism Using Single-Subject Experimentation and Group Analysis Methods," *Nursing Research* 54 (2005): 22–32.

20. Jacinta Bronte-Tinkew, Mary Burkhauser, and Allison J. R. Mertz, "Elements of Promising Practices in Fatherhood Programs: Evidence-based Research Findings on Interventions for Fathers," *Fathering* 10 (2012): 6–30.

21. Ibid.; Marsiglio and Roy, *Nurturing Dads.*

22. Marsiglio and Roy, *Nurturing Dads*; see also Gayle Kaufman, *Superdads: How Fathers Balance Work and Family in the 21st Century* (New York: New York University Press, 2013); Jeremy A. Smith, *The Daddy Shift: How Stay-at-Home-Dads, Breadwinning Moms, and Shared Parenting Are Transforming the American Family* (Boston: Beacon, 2009).

23. Bronte-Tinkew, Burkhauser, and Mertz, "Elements of Promising Practices in Fatherhood Programs."

24. Marsiglio, *Men on a Mission.*

25. For suggestions on how health care providers can treat men as "coproducers" of their health, see Demetrius J. Porche, "Engaging Men As Coproducers in Health Care," *American Journal of Men's Health* 9, no. 2 (2015): 93.

26. Justin J. Hendricks, Heidi Steinour, Heidi, William Marsiglio, and Deepika Kulkarni, "Magazine Depictions of Fathers' Involvement in Children's Health: A Content Analysis," in *Deconstructing Dads: Changing Images of Fathers in Popular Culture*, ed. Laura Tropp and Janice Kelly (Lanham, MD: Lexington Books, 2016), 143–163.

BIBLIOGRAPHY

Adams, Kenneth F., Arthur Schatzkin, Tamara B. Harris, Victor Kipnis, Traci Mouw, Rachel Ballard-Barbash, Albert Hollenbeck, and Michael F. Litzmann. "Overweight, Obesity, and Mortality in a Large Prospective Cohort of Persons 50 to 71 Years Old." *New England Journal of Medicine* 355(8) (2006): 763–778.

Ajani, U. A., P. A. Lutofuo, J. M. Gaziano, I. M. Lee, A. Spelsberg, J. E. Buring, W. C. Willett, and J. E. Manson. "Body Mass Index and Mortality among US Male Physicians." *Annals of Epidemiology* 14 (2004): 731–739.

Allen, Sarah M., and Alan J. Hawkins. "Maternal Gatekeeping: Mothers' Beliefs and Behaviors That Inhibit Greater Father Involvement in Family Work." *Journal of Marriage and Family* 61, no. 1 (1999): 199–212.

Al-Yagon, Michal. "Fathers' Emotional Resources and Children's Socioemotional and Behavioral Adjustment among Children with Learning Disabilities." *Journal of Child Family Studies* 20 (2011): 569–584.

American Academy of Pediatrics. "Breastfeeding and the Use of Human Milk." *Pediatrics* 115 (2005): 496–506.

Anderson, Eric, and Edward Kian. "Examining Media Contestation of Masculinity and Head Trauma in the National Football League." *Men and Masculinities* 15 (2012): 152–173.

Artis, Julie E. "Breastfeed at Your Own Risk." *Contexts* 8 (2009): 28–34.

Aumann, Kerstin, Ellen Galinsky, and Kenneth Matos. *The New Male Mystique.* New York: Families and Work Institute, 2011.

Barr, Donald A. *Health Disparities in the United States: Social Class, Race, Ethnicity, and Health.* Baltimore, MD: Johns Hopkins University Press, 2008.

Barzansky, Barbara, and Sylvia I. Etzel. "Medical Schools in the United States, 2013–2014." *JAMA* 312, no. 22 (2014): 2419–2426.

Bazargan, Mohsen, Marian Makar, Shahrzad Bazargan-Hejazi, Chizobam Ani, and Kenneth E. Wolf. "Preventive, Lifestyle, and Personal Health Behaviors among Physicians." *Academic Psychiatry* 33 (2009): 289–295.

Bonsall, Aaron. "Fathering Occupations: An Analysis of Narrative Accounts of Fathering Children with Special Needs." *Journal of Occupational Science* 21(4) (2014): 504–518.

Boyle, Coleen A., Sheree Boulet, Laura A. Schieve, Robin A. Cohen, Stephen J. Blumberg, Marshalyn Yeargin-Allsopp, Susanna Visser, and Michael D. Kogan. "Trends in the Prevalence of Developmental Disabilities in US Children, 1997–2008." *Pediatrics* 127 (2011): 1034–1042.

Brody, Amanda C., and Leigh Ann Simmons. "Family Resiliency during Childhood Cancer: The Father's Perspective." *Journal of Pediatric Oncology Nursing* 24(3) (2007): 152–165.

Brooks, Samantha K., Clare Gerada, and Trudie Chalder. "Review of Literature on the Mental Health of Doctors: Are Specialist Services Needed?" *Journal of Mental Health* 20 (2011): 146–156.

Bronte-Tinkew, Jacinta, Mary Burkhauser, and Allison J. R. Mertz. "Elements of Promising Practices in Fatherhood Programs: Evidence-Based Research Findings on Interventions for Fathers." *Fathering* 10 (2012): 6–30.

Broom, Alex, and Philip Tovey. *Men's Health: Body, Identity, and Social Context.* Chichester, West Sussex, UK: Wiley-Blackwell, 2009.

Brophy, Sinead, Anwen Rees, Gareth Knox, Julien Baker, and Non E. Thomas. "Child Fitness and Father's BMI Are Important Factors in Childhood Obesity: A School-Based Cross-Sectional Study." *Www.Plosone.Org* 7, no. 5 (2012), E36597: 1–7.

Brown, Linda Keller, and Kay Mussell. "Introduction." In Ethnic and Regional Foodways in the United States: The Performance of Group Identity, ed. Linda Keller Brown and Kay Mussell, 3–15. Knoxville: The University of Tennessee Press, 1984.

Casper, M. J. *The Making of the Unborn Patient: A Social Anatomy of Fetal Surgery.* New Brunswick, NJ: Rutgers University Press, 1998.

Clarke, Juanne N. "Father's Home Health Care Work When a Child Has Cancer: I'm Her Dad, I Have to Do It." *Men and Masculinities* 7, no. 4 (2005): 385–404.

Coakley, Jay. "The Good Father: Parental Expectations and Youth Sports." *Leisure Studies* 25 (2006): 153–163.

Coffield, Edward, Allison J. Nihiser, Bettylou Sherry, and Christina D. Economos. "Shape Up Somerville: Change in Parent Body Mass Indexes during a Child-Targeted, Community-Based Environmental Change Intervention." *American Journal of Public Health* 105, no. 2 (2015): E83–389.

Cohen, Diana T. *Iron Dads: Managing Work, Family, and Endurance Sport Identities.* New Brunswick, NJ: Rutgers University Press, 2016.

Coleman, William L., and Craig Garfield, and American Academy of Pediatrics, Committee on Psychosocial Aspects of Child and Family Health. "Fathers and Pediatricians: Enhancing Men's Roles in the Care and Development of Their Children." *Pediatrics* 113, no. 5 (2004): 1406–1411.

Cortese, Samuele, Maria Olazagasti, Rachel Klein, F. Castellanos, Ericka Proal, and Salvatore Mannuzza. "Obesity in Men with Childhood ADHD: A 33-Year Controlled, Prospective, Follow-Up Study." *Pediatrics* 131 (2013): 1731–1738.

Courtenay, W. H. "Constructions of Masculinity and Their Influence on Men's Well-Being: A Theory of Gender and Health." *Social Science and Medicine* 50 (2000): 1385–1401.

———. *Dying to Be Men: Psychosocial, Environmental, and Biobehavioral Directions in Promoting the Health of Men and Boys.* New York: Routledge, 2011.

Cox, D. N., B. K. Wittman, M. Hess, A. G. Ross, J. Lind, and S. Lindahl. "The Psychological Impact of Diagnostic Ultrasound." *Obstetrics and Gynecology* 70, no. 5 (1987): 673–676.

Crossen, Eric J., Brenna Lewis, and Benjamin D. Hoffman. "Preventing Gun Injuries in Children." *Pediatrics in Review* 36 (2015): 43–51.

Daniels, Cynthia R. *The Science and Politics of Male Reproduction.* Oxford: Oxford University Press, 2006.

Davis, Kevin C., W. Douglas Evans, and Kian Kamyab. "Effectiveness of a National Campaign to Promote Parent-Child Communication About Sex." *Health Education & Behavior* 40 (2013): 97–106.

de St. Aubin, Ed, Dan P. Mcadams, and Kim Tae-Chang. *The Generative Society: Caring for Future Generations.* Washington, DC: American Psychological Association, 2004.

Deutsch, Jonathan, and Rachel D. Saks. *Jewish American Food Culture.* Westport, CT: Greenwood, 2008.

Doucet, Andrea. *Do Men Mother? Fathering, Care, and Domestic Responsibility.* Toronto: University of Toronto Press, 2006.

Draper, Jan. "'It Was a Real Good Show': The Ultrasound Scan, Fathers, and the Power of Visual Knowledge." *Sociology of Health & Illness* 24 (2002): 771–795.

Drug Policy Alliance. "Healing a Broken System: Veterans Battling Addiction and Incarceration." Issue brief, November 4, 2009. https://www.phoenixhouse.org/wp-content/uploads/2010/12/DPA_IssueBrief_Veterans.pdf. Accessed February 14, 2016.

Duvdevany, Ilana, Eli Buchbinder, and Ilanit Yaacov. "Accepting Disability: The Parenting Experience of Fathers with Spinal Cord Injury (SCI)." *Qualitative Health Research* 18, no. 8 (2008): 1021–1033.

Edleson, J. L. "Emerging Responses to Children Exposed to Domestic Violence." Harrisburg, PA: Vawnet, a Project of the National Resource Center on Domestic Violence/Pennsylvania Coalition against Domestic Violence, 2006. http://www.vawnet.org. Accessed March 15, 2014.

Edward, Karen-Leigh, David Castle, Cally Mills, Leigh Davis, and June Casey. "An Integrative Review of Paternal Depression." *American Journal of Men's Health* 9 (2015): 26–34.

Elder, Jennifer H., Susan O. Donaldson, John Kairalla, Gregory Valcante, Roxanna Bendixen, Richard Ferdig, Erica Self, Jeffrey Walker, Christina Palau, and Michele Serrano. "In-Home Training for Fathers of Children with Autism: A Follow Up Study and Evaluation of Four Individual Training Components." *Journal of Child and Family Studies* 20 (2011): 263–271.

Elder, Jennifer H., Gregory Valcante, Hassein Yarandi, Deborah White, and Timothy H. Elder. "Evaluating in-Home Training for Fathers of Children with Autism Using Single-Subject Experimentation and Group Analysis Methods." *Nursing Research* 54 (2005): 22–32.

Erikson, Erik H. *Life History and the Historical Moment.* New York: Norton, 197.

Fagan, Jay, and Marina Barnett. "The Relationship between Maternal Gatekeeping, Paternal Competence, Mothers' Attitudes About the Father Role, and Father Involvement." *Journal of Family Issues* 24 (2003):1020–1043.

Feinberg, Mark E. "Coparenting and the Transition to Parenthood: A Framework for Prevention." *Clinical Child and Family Psychology Review* 5 (2002): 173–195.

———. "The Internal Structure and Ecological Context of Coparenting: A Framework for Research and Intervention." *Parenting: Science and Practice* 3 (2003): 95–131.

Finkelhor, David, Heather Turner, Richard Ormrod, Sherry L. Hamby. "Violence, Abuse, and Crime Exposure in a National Sample of Children and Youth." *Pediatrics* 124 (2009): 1411–1423.

Frank, Erica, Holly Biola, and Carol A. Burnett. "Mortality Rates and Causes among U.S. Physicians." *American Journal of Preventive Medicine* 19 (2000): 155–159.

Fraser, Josephine, Helen Skouteris, Marita Mccabe, Lina A. Ricciardelli, Jeannette Milgrom, and Louise Baur. "Paternal Influences on Children's Weight Gain: A Systematic Review." *Fathering* 9 (2011): 252–267.

Freeman, E., R. Fletcher, C. E. Collins, P. J. Morgan, T. Burrows, and R. Callister. "Preventing and Treating Childhood Obesity: Time to Target Fathers." *International Journal of Obesity* 36 (2012): 12–15.

Fujiwara, Takeo, Makiko Okuyama, and Kunihiko Takahashi. "Paternal Involvement in Childcare and Unintentional Injury of Young Children: A Population-Based Cohort Study in Japan." *International Journal of Epidemiology* 39 (2010): 588–597.

Garfield, Craig F. "Fathers and the Well-Child Visit." *Pediatrics* 117 (2006): 637–645.

Garfield, Craig F., and Anthony J. Isacco III. "Urban Fathers' Involvement in Their Child's Health and Healthcare." *Psychology of Men & Masculinity* 13 (2012): 32–48.

Gillman, M. "Family Dinner and Diet Quality among Older Children and Adolescents." *Archives of Family Medicine* 9 (2000): 235–240.

Gilman, Stephan E., Richard Rende, Julie Boergers, David. B. Abrams, Stephen L. Buka, Melissa A. Clark, Suzanne M. Colby, Brian Hitsman, Alessandra N. Kazura, Lewis P. Lipsitt, Elizabeth E. Lloyd-Richardson. Michelle L. Rogers, Cassandra A. Stanton, Laura R. Stroud, and Raymond S. Niaura. 2009. "Parental Smoking and Adolescent Smoking Initiation: An Intergenerational Perspective on Tobacco Control." *Pediatrics* 123, no. 2 (2009): E274–E281. doi10.1542/Peds. 2008–2251.

Giorgianni, Salvatore. J., [primary], Thomas Berger, Jean Bonhomme, Eric D. Bothwell, Armin Brott, Paris D. Butler, Olivia Casey, et al. "A Framework for Advancing the Overall Health and Wellness of America's Boys and Men." Position paper issued by the Men's Health Braintrust, Dialogue on Men's Health, March 2013. http://www .menshealthnetwork.org/library/Dialogue1.pdf.

Glaze, Lauren E., and Laura M. Maruschak. "Parents in Prison and Their Minor Children." Bureau of Justice Statistics Special Report, revised March 30, 2010. http:// www.bjs.gov/content/pub/pdf/pptmc.pdf. Accessed September 25, 2015.

Goldberg, Herb. *The Hazards of Being Male: Surviving the Myth of Masculine Privilege.* Ojai, CA: Iconoclassics, 2009.

Golub, Andrew, Peter Vazan, Alexander S. Bennett, and Hilary J. Liberty. "Unmet Need for Treatment of Substance Use Disorders and Serious Psychological Distress among Veterans: A Nationwide Analysis Using the NSDUH." *Military Medicine* 178 (2013): 107–114.

Gottzén, Lucas, and Tamar Kremer-Sadlik. "Fatherhood and Youth Sports: A Balancing Act between Care and Expectations." *Gender & Society* 26 (2012): 639–664.

Gustafson, Sabrina L., and Ryan E. Rhodes. "Parental Correlates of Physical Activity in Children and Early Adolescents." *Sports Medicine* 36 (2006): 79–97.

Hallberg, Ann-Christine, Anders Beckman, and Anders Håkansson. "Many Fathers Visit the Child Health Care Centre, but Few Take Part in Parents' Groups." *Journal of Child Health Care* 14, no. 3 (2010): 296–303.

Hamby, Sherry, David Finkelhor, Heather Turner, and Richard Ormrod. "Children's Exposure to Intimate Partner Violence and Other Family Violence: Nationally Representative Rates Among US Youth." OJJDP *Juvenile Justice Bulletin-NCJ* 232272, October 2011, 1–12. Washington, DC: Government Printing Office. Available at http://scholars.unh.edu/cgi/viewcontent.cgi?article=1026&context=ccrc.

Harrington, Brad, Fred Van Deusen, and Beth Humberd. *The New Dad: Caring, Committed, and Conflicted.* Boston: Boston College Center for Work and Family, 2011.

Harrington, Brad, Fred Van Deusen, and Jamie Ladge. 2010. *The New Dad: Exploring Fatherhood within a Career Context.* Boston: Boston College Center for Work and Family, 2010.

Hartling, Lisa, Andrea Milne, Lisa Tjosvold, Dawn Wrightson, Jennifer Gallivan, and Amand S. Newton. "A Systematic Review of Interventions to Support Siblings of Children with Chronic Illness or Disability." *Journal of Paediatrics and Child Health.* 50 (2014): E26-E38. doi:10.1111/J.1440–1754.2010.01771.x.

Hendricks, Justin J., Heidi Steinour, Heidi, William Marsiglio, and Deepika Kulkarni. "Magazine Depictions of Fathers' Involvement in Children's Health: A Content Analysis." In *Deconstructing Dads: Changing Images of Fathers in Popular Culture*, edited by Laura Tropp and Janice Kelly, 143–163. Lanham, MD: Lexington, 2016.

Hill, David L. *Dad to Dad: Parenting Like a Pro: Expert Advice, Guidance, and Insight from a Pediatrician-Dad.* Elk Grove, IL: American Academy of Pediatrics, 2012.

Hill, Karalyn, Aiveen Higgins, Martin Dempster, and Anthony Mccarthy. "Fathers' Views and Understanding of Their Roles in Families with a Child with Acute Lymphoblastic Leukaemia: An Interpretative Phenomenological Analysis." *Journal of Health Psychology* 14, no. 8 (2009): 1268–1280.

Hosegood, Victorica, Linda Richter, and Lynda Clarke. "'. . . I Should Maintain a Healthy Life Now and Not Just Live As I Please . . .': Men's Health and Fatherhood in Rural South Africa." *American Journal of Men's Health* 1–12 (2015). doi:10.1177/1557988315586440.

Hovey, Judith K. "Differences in Parenting Needs of Fathers of Children with Chronic Conditions Related to Family Income." *Journal of Child Health Care* 10, no. 1 (2006): 43–54.

———. "The Needs of Fathers Parenting Children with Chronic Conditions." *Journal of Pediatric Oncology Nursing* 20, no. 5 (2003): 245–251.

Humberd, Beth, Jamie J. Ladge, and Brad Harrington. "The 'New' Dad: Navigating Fathering Identity within Organizational Contexts." *Journal of Business and Psychology* 30 (2015): 249–266.

Interagency Youth Working Group. "Mobile Technology for Health." Youth Lens on Reproductive Health and HIV/AIDS, no. 38. Research Triangle Park, NC, 2013. https://www.iywg.org/sites/iywg/files/yl_38_mobiletech.pdf. Accessed February 14, 2016.

Jamal, Ahmed, Israel T. Agaku, Erin O'Conner, Brian A. King, John B. Kenemer, and Linda Neff. "Current Cigarette Smoking among Adults—United States, 2005–2013." Centers for Disease Control and Prevention, *Morbidity and Mortality Weekly Report* 63, no. 47 (2014).

Janer, Zilkia. *Latino Food Culture*. Westport, CT: Greenwood, 2008.

Jenks, Elaine Bass. "Explaining Disability: Parents' Stories of Raising Children with Visual Impairments in a Sighted World." *Journal of Contemporary Ethnography* 34 (2005): 143–169.

Johnson, Martin P., and John E. Puddifoot. "Miscarriage: Is Vividness of Visual Imagery a Factor in the Grief Reaction of the Partner?" *British Journal of Health Psychology* 3 (1998): 137–146.

Jordan, Brigitte. "Authoritative Knowledge and Its Construction." In *Childbirth and Authoritative Knowledge: Cross-Cultural Perspectives*, edited by Robbie E. Davis-Floyd and Carolyn F. Sargent, 55–79. Berkeley: University of California Press, 1997.

Jordan, Pamela L., and Virginia R. Wall. "Breastfeeding and Fathers: Illuminating the Darker Side." *Birth* 17 (1990): 210–213.

Kaufman, Gayle. *Superdads: How Fathers Balance Work and Family in the 21st Century*. New York: New York University Press, 2013.

Kelly, Joe. *Dads and Daughters: How to Inspire, Understand, and Support Your Daughter When She's Growing Up So Fast*. New York: Broadway Books, 2002.

Khan, Shama, Ahmed A. Arif, Jamie N. Laditka, and Elizabeth F. Racine. "Prenatal Exposure to Secondhand Smoke May Increase the Risk of Postpartum Depressive Symptoms." *Journal of Public Health* (2015). doi:10.1093/Pubmed/Fdv083.

Kilkey, Majella, and Harriet Clarke. "Disabled Men and Fathering: Opportunities and Constraints." *Community, Work & Family* 13 (2010): 127–146.

Kimmel, Michael. *Guyland: The Inner World of Young Men*. New York: HarperCollins, 2008.

Kitzmann, Katherine M., Noni K. Gaylord, Aimee R. Holt, and Erin D. Kenny. "Child Witnesses to Domestic Violence: A Meta-Analytic Review." *Journal of Consulting and Clinical Psychology* 71 (2003): 339–352.

Kramer, Zachary A. "Of Meat and Manhood." *Washington University Law Review* 89 (2011): 287–322.

Leavitt, Judith Walzer. *Make Room for Daddy: The Journey from Waiting Room to Birthing Room*. Chapel Hill: University of North Carolina Press, 2009.

Leonardi-Bee, Jo, John Britton, and Andrea Venn. "Secondhand Smoke and Adverse Fetal Outcomes in Nonsmoking Pregnant Women: A Meta Analysis." *Pediatrics* 127, no. 4 (2011): 734–741.

Lesser, Lenard I., Deborah A. Cohen, and Robert H. Brook. "Changing Eating Habits for the Medical Profession." *JAMA* 308 (2012): 983–984.

Levant, Ronald. F., David. J. Wimer, Christine M. Williams, K. Bryant Smalley, and Delilah Noronha. "The Relationships between Masculinity Variables, Health Risk Behaviors, and Attitudes toward Seeking Psychological Help." *International Journal of Men's Health* 8 (2009): 3–21.

Levi, Jeffrey, Laura M. Segal, Rebecca St. Laurent, and Jack Rayburn. *State of Obesity Report*. Rep. Trust for America's Health. Robert Wood Johnson Foundation, 2014. http://www.rwjf.org/content/dam/farm/reports/reports/2014/rwjf414829. Accessed May 19, 2015.

Louv, Richard. *The Last Child in the Woods: Saving Our Children from Nature-Deficit Disorder*. Chapel Hill, NC: Algonquin Books, 2008.

———. *The Nature Principle: Reconnecting with Life in a Virtual Age*. Chapel Hill, NC: Algonquin Books, 2012.

Macdonald, Elaine E., and Richard P. Hastings. "Fathers of Children with Developmental Disabilities." In *The Role of the Father in Child Development*, 5th ed., edited by Michael E. Lamb, 486–516. Hoboken, NJ: Wiley, 2010.

Madden, Mary, Amanda Lenhart, Maeve Duggan, Sandra Cortesi, and Urs Gasser. "Teens and Technology." Washington, DC: Pew Research Center, 2013. http://www.pewinternet.org/reports/2013/teens-and-tech.aspx. Accessed September 2, 2013.

Marcus, Steven C., and Mark Olfson. "National Trends in the Treatment for Depression from 1998 to 2007." *Archives of General Psychiatry* 67 (2010): 1265–1273.

Marsiglio, William. "Being a Dad, Studying Fathers: Personal Reflections." In *Papa, PhD: Essays on Fatherhood by Men in the Academy*, edited by Mary Ruth Marotte, Paige Martin Reynolds, and Ralph James Savarese, 135–140. New Brunswick, NJ: Rutgers University Press, 2011.

———. "Healthy Dads, Healthy Kids." *Contexts* 8 (2009): 22–27.

———"Making Males Mindful of Their Sexual and Procreative Identities: Using Self-Narratives in Field Settings." *Perspectives on Sexual and Reproductive Health* 35 (2003): 229–233.

———. *Men on a Mission: Valuing Youth Work in Our Communities*. Baltimore, MD: Johns Hopkins University Press, 2008.

———. *Stepdads: Stories of Hope, Love, and Repair*. Lanham, MD: Rowman & Littlefield, 2004.

Marsiglio, William, and Sally Hutchinson. *Sex, Men, and Babies: Stories of Awareness and Responsibility*. New York: New York University Press, 2002.

Marsiglio, William, and Kevin Roy. *Nurturing Dads: Social Initiatives for Contemporary Fatherhood*. ASA Rose Monograph Series. New York: Russell Sage Foundation, 2012.

Marsiglio, William, Kevin Roy, and Greer Litton Fox. "Conceptualizing Situated Fatherhood: A Spatially-Sensitive and Social Approach." In *Situated Fathering: A Focus on Physical and Social Spaces*, edited by William Marsiglio, Kevin Roy, and Greer Litton Fox, 3–26. Lanham, MD: Rowman & Littlefield, 2005.

McNeill, Ted. "Fathers of Children with a Chronic Health Condition: Beyond Gender Stereotypes." *Men and Masculinities* 9. no. 4 (2007): 409–424.

Merlo, Lisa J., and Mark S. Gold. "Prescription Opioid Abuse and Dependence among Physicians: Hypotheses and Treatment." *Harvard Review of Psychiatry* 16 (2008): 181–194.

Messner, Michael. *It's All for the Kids: Gender, Family, and Youth Sports*. Berkeley: University of California Press, 2009.

———. "The Life of a Man's Seasons: Male Identity in the Life Course of the Athlete." In *Changing Men: New Directions in Research on Men and Masculinity*, edited by Michael S. Kimmel, 54–67. Thousand Oaks, CA: Sage, 1987.

———. "Masculinities and Athletic Careers." *Gender & Society* 3 (1989):71–88.

Metzl, Jonathan M. 2010. "Why 'Against Health'?" In *Against Health: How Health Became the New Morality*, edited by Jonathan M. Mentz and Anna Kirland, 1–14. New York: New York University Press, 2010.

Metzl, Jonathan M., and Anna Kirland, eds. *Against Health: How Health Became the New Morality*. New York: New York University Press, 2010.

Miller, Tina. "'It's a Triangle That's Difficult to Square': Men's Intentions and Practices Around Caring, Work and First-time Fatherhood." *Fathering* 8. no. 3 (2010): 362–378.

Mojibyan, Mahideyeh, Mehran Karimi, Reza Bidaki, and Asghar Zare. "Exposure to Second-Hand Smoke during Pregnancy and Preterm Delivery." *International Journal of High Risk Behaviors and Addiction* 1, no. 4 (2013): 149–153.

Moola, Fiola. J. "This Is the Best Fatal Illness That You Can Have: Contrasting and Comparing the Experiences of Parenting Youth with Cystic Fibrosis and Congenital Heart Disease." *Qualitative Health Research* 22 (2012): 212–225.

Morgan, Philip J., Clare E. Collins, Ronald C. Plotnikoff, Robin Callister, Tracy Burrows, Richard Fletcher, Anthony D. Okely, Myles D. Young, Andrew Miller, Adam B. Lloyd, Alyce T. Cook, Joel Cruickshank, Kristen Saunders, and David R. Lubans. "The 'Healthy Dads, Healthy Kids' Community Randomized Controlled Trial: A Community-Based Healthy Lifestyle Program for Fathers and Their Children." *Preventive Medicine* 61 (2014): 90–99.

Nepomnyaschy, Lenna, and Louis Donnelly. "Father Involvement and Childhood Injuries." *Journal of Marriage and Family* 77 (2015): 628–646.

Newbould, Jennifer, Felicity Smith, and Sally-Anne Francis. "'I'm Fine Doing It on My Own': Partnership between Young People and Their Parents in the Management of Medication for Asthma and Diabetes." *Journal of Child Health Care* 12 (2008): 116–128.

Nielsen, Linda. *Father-Daughter Relationships: Contemporary Research and Issues*. New York: Routledge, 2012.

Olsen, Lisa L., John L. Oliffe, Marianna Brussoni, and Genevieve Creighton. "Fathers' Views on Their Financial Situations, Father-Child Activities, and Preventing Child Injuries." *American Journal of Men's Health* 9 (2015): 15–25.

Ortiz, Robert W., Tim Green, and Hee-Jeong Lim. "Families and Home Computer Use: Exploring Parent Perceptions of the Importance of Current Technology." *Urban Education* 46. no. 2 (2011): 202–215.

Paulson, James F., and Sharnail D. Bazemore. "Prenatal and Postpartum Depression in Fathers and Its Association with Maternal Depression: A Meta-Analysis." *JAMA* 303 (2010): 1961–1969.

Petchesky, Rosalind Pollack. "Foetal Images: The Power of Visual Culture in the Politics of Reproduction." *Feminist Studies* 13. no. 2 (1987): 263–292.

Plantin, Lars, Adepeju Aderemi Olukoya, and Pernilla Ny. "Positive Health Outcomes of Fathers' Involvement in Pregnancy and Childbirth Paternal Support: A Scope Study Literature Review." *Fathering* 9 (2011): 87–102.

Pleck, Joseph H. "Paternal Involvement: Revised Conceptualization and Theoretical Linkages with Child Outcomes." In *the Role of the Father in Child Development*. 5th ed. Edited by Michael E. Lamb, 67–107. Hoboken, NJ: Wiley, 2010.

Pleck, Joseph H., and Brian P. Masciadrelli. "Paternal Involvement by U.S. Residential Fathers: Levels, Sources, and Consequences." In *The Role of the Father in Child Development*, 4th ed., edited by Michael E. Lamb. Hoboken, NJ: Wiley, 2004.

Pollack, William. *Real Boys: Rescuing Our Sons from the Myths of Boyhood.* New York: Henry Holt, 1999.

Porche, Demetrius J. "Engaging Men As Coproducers in Health Care." *American Journal of Men's Health* 9. no. 2 (2015): 93.

Presley, Christal. *Thirty Days with My Father: Finding Peace from Wartime PTSD.* Deerfield Beach, FL: Health Communications, 2012.

Ramchandani, Paul, Alan Stein, Thomas G. O'Conner, and the ALSPAC Study Team. 2015. "Paternal Depression in the Postnatal Period and Child Development: A Prospective Population Study." *Lancet* 365 (2015): 2201–2205.

Richardson, Noel, and Paula Carroll. "National Men's Health Policy 2008–2013: Working with Men in Ireland to Achieve Optimum Health & Wellbeing." Dublin, Ireland: Department of Health and Children, Minister for Health and Children, 2008.

Rippeyoung, Phyllis L. F., and Mary C. Noonan. "Breastfeeding and the Gendering of Infant Care." In *Beyond Health, Beyond Choice: Breastfeeding Constraints and Realities*, edited by B. L. Hausman, P. Hall Smith, and M. Labbok, 133–143. New Brunswick, NJ: Rutgers University Press, 2012.

———. "Is Breastfeeding Truly Cost Free? Income Consequences of Breastfeeding for Women." *American Sociological Review* 77 (2012): 244–267.

Rogers, Richard. "Beasts, Burgers and Hummers: Meat and the Crisis of Masculinity in Contemporary Television Advertisements." *Environmental Communication* 2 (2008): 281–301.

Roman, Pawlak, Ding Qin, and Sovyanhadi Marta. "Pregnancy Outcome and Breastfeeding Pattern among Vegans, Vegetarians, and Non-Vegetarians." *Eliven: Journal of Dietetics Research and Nutrition* 1 (2014): 1–4.

Rothman, Barbara Katz. *The Tentative Pregnancy: Amniocentesis and the Sexual Politics of Motherhood.* London: Pandora, 1994.

Rozin, Paul, Julia M. Hormes, Myles S. Faith, and Brian Wansink. "Is Meat Male? A Quantitative Multi-Method Framework to Establish Metaphoric Relationships." *Journal of Consumer Research* 39 (2012): 629–643.

Ryan, Caitlin. "Helping Families Support Their Lesbian, Gay, Bisexual, and Transgender (LGBT) Children." Washington, DC: National Center for Cultural Competence, Georgetown University Center for Child and Human Development, 2009.

Sabo, Donald, and David F. Gordon. *Men's Health and Illness: Gender, Power, and the Body*. Thousand Oaks, CA: Sage, 1995.

Sabo, Donald, and Phil Veliz. *Go Out and Play: Youth Sports in America*. East Meadow, NY: Women's Sports Foundation, 2008.

Samson, André, E. Tomiak, J. Dimillo, R. Lavigne, S. Miles, M. Choquette, P. Chakraborty, and P. Jacob. "The Lived Experience of Hope among Parents of a Child with Duchenne Muscular Dystrophy: Perceiving the Human Being Beyond the Illness." *Chronic Illness* 5 (2009): 103–114.

Samuels, Debra. "Food-Savvy Dads at the Stove." *Boston Globe*, June 16, 2015. https://www.bostonglobe.com/lifestyle/food-dining/2015/06/16/food-savvy-dads-stove/0aw6ioxdqos71byzioxmem/story.html. Accessed June 17, 2015.

Sayers, Steven L. "Family Reintegration Difficulties and Couples Therapy for Military Veterans and Their Spouses." *Cognitive and Behavioral Practice* 18 (2011): 108–119.

Schoppe-Sullivan, Sarah J., Geoffrey L. Brown, Elizabeth A. Cannon, Sarah C. Mangelsdorf, and Margaret Szewczyk Sokolowski. "Maternal Gatekeeping, Coparenting Quality, and Fathering Behavior in Families with Infants." *Journal of Family Psychology* 22 (2008): 389–398.

Schwebel, David C., and Carl M. Brezausek. "How Do Mothers and Fathers Influence Pediatric Injury Risk in Middle Childhood?" *Journal of Pediatric Psychology* 35 (2010): 806–813.

Seligson, Hannah. "Don't Call Him Mom, or an Imbecile." *New York Times*, February 23, 2012. http://www.nytimes.com/2013/02/24/business/fathers-seek-advertising-that-does-not-ridicule.html?pagewanted=all&_r=0. Accessed March 17, 2014.

Senay, Emily, and Rob Waters. *From Boys to Men: A Women's Guide to the Health of Husbands, Partners, Sons, Fathers, and Brothers*. New York: Scribner, 2004.

Silvern, Louise, Jane Karyl, Lynn Waelde, William F. Hodges, Joanna Starek, Elizabeth Heidt, and Kyung Min. "Retrospective Reports of Parental Partner Abuse: Relationships to Depression, Trauma Symptoms, and Self-Esteem among College Students." *Journal of Family Violence* 10 (1995): 177–202.

Skolnikoff, Jessica, and Robert Engvall. *Youth Athletes, Couch Potatoes, and Helicopter Parents: The Productivity of Play*. Lanham, MD: Rowman & Littlefield, 2014.

Sobal, Jeffrey. "Men, Meat, and Marriage: Models of Masculinity." *Food and Foodways* 13 (2005): 135–158.

Stein, R., L. Epstein, H. Raynor, C. Kilanowski, and R. Paluc. "The Influence of Parenting Change on Pediatric Weight Control." *Obesity* 13 (2005): 1749–1755.

Sterken, David J. "Uncertainty and Coping in Fathers of Children with Cancer." *Journal of Pediatric Oncology Nursing* 13, no. 2 (1996): 81–88.

Stewart, Susan D. "Disneyland Dads, Disneyland Moms? How Nonresident Parents Spend Time with Absent Children." *Journal of Family Issues* 20 (1999): 539–556.

Taylor, Janelle S. "The Public Foetus and the Family Car: From Abortion Politics to a Volvo Advertisement." *Science As Culture* 3, no. 17 (1993): 601–618.

Thomas, William I., and Dorothy Swain Thomas. *The Child in America: Behavior Problems and Programs*. New York: Knopf, 1928.

Tiedje, Linda Beth, and Cynthia Darling-Fisher. "Promoting Father-Friendly Health-care." *MCN* 28 (2003): 350–359.

Tonstad, Serena, Terry Butler, Ru Yan, and Gary E. Fraser. "Type of Vegetarian Diet, Body Weight, and Prevalence of Type 2 Diabetes." *Diabetes Care* 32 (2009): 791–796.

U.S. Bureau of the Census. *Facts for Feature. Father's Day: June 21, 2105.* U.S. Bureau of the Census, Facts for Features, 2015. http://census.gov/content/dam/Census/newsroom/facts-for-features/2015/cb15-ff11.pdf.

Veatch, Robert M. "Models for Ethical Medicine in a Revolutionary Age." *Hastings Center Report* 2 (1972): 5–7.

Visser, S., M. Danielson, R. H. Bitsko, J. R. Kogan, M. D., R. M. Ghandour, R. Perou, and S. J. Blumberg. "Trends in the Parent-Report of Health Care Provider-Diagnosis and Medication Treatment for ADHD Disorder: United States, 2003–2011." *Journal of the American Academy of Child and Adolescent Psychiatry* 53, no. 1 (2014): 34–46.

Vuolo, Mike, and Jeremy Staff. "Parent and Child Cigarette Use: A Longitudinal Multi-generational Study." *Pediatrics* 132 (2013): 1–10.

Wake, Milissa, Jan M. Nicholson, Pollyanna Hardy, and Katherine Smith. "Pre-schooler Obesity and Parenting Styles of Mothers and Fathers: Australian National Population Study." *Pediatrics* 120, no. 6 (2007): E1520–E1527.

Walker, Alexis J., and Lori A. McGraw. "Who Is Responsible for Responsible Father-ing?" *Journal of Marriage and Family* 62 (2000): 563–570.

Wang, Rong, Suzanne M. Bianchi, and Sara B. Raley. "Teenagers' Internet Use and Fam-ily Rules: A Research Note." *Journal of Marriage and Family* 67 (2005): 1249–1258.

Ware, Jane, and H. Hitesh Raval. "A Qualitative Investigation of Fathers' Experiences of Looking After a Child with a Life-Limiting Illness, in Process and Retrospect." *Clinical Child Psychology and Psychiatry* 12 (2007): 549–565.

Widarsson, Margareta, Gabriella Engsröm, Tanja Tydén, Pranee Lundberg, and Lena Marmstål Hammar. "'Paddling Upstream': Fathers' Involvement during Pregnancy As Described by Expectant Fathers and Mothers." *Journal of Clinical Nursing* 24 (2015): 1059–1068.

Wilk, Joshua E., Paul D. Bliese, Paul Y. Kim, Jeffrey L. Thomas, Dennis Mcgurk, and Charles W. Hoge. "Relationship of Combat Experiences to Alcohol Misuse among U.S. Soldiers Returning from the Iraq War." *Drug and Alcohol Dependence* 108 (2009): 115–121.

Wisner, Katherine L., Dorothy K. Y. Sit, Mary C. Mcshea, David M. Rizzo, Rebecca A. Zoretich, Carolyn L. Hughes, Heather F. Eng, James F. Luther, Stephen R. Wis-niewski, Michelle L. Costantino, Andrea L. Confer, Eydie L. Moses-Kolko, Chris-topher S. Famy, and Barbara H. Hanusa. "Onset Timing, Thoughts of Self-Harm, and Diagnoses in Postpartum Women with Screen-Positive Depression Findings." *JAMA Psychiatry* 70, no. 5 (2013): 490–498. doi:10.1001/jamapsychiatry.2013.87.

Witt, Edward A., Adam J. Massman, and Linda A. Jackson. "Trends in Youth's Video-game Playing, Overall Computer Use, and Communication Technology Use: The Impact of Self-Esteem and the Big Five Personality Factors." *Computers in Human Behavior* 27 (2011): 763–769.

Wolf, Jacqueline H. "Low Breastfeeding Rates and Public Health in the United States." *American Journal of Public Health* 93 (2003): 2000–2010.

Wolf, Joan B. "Is Breast Really Best? Risk and Total Motherhood in the National Breastfeeding Awareness Campaign." *Journal of Health Politics, Policy, and Law* 32 (2007): 596–636.

Zvara, Bharathi, Sarah J. Schoppe-Sullivan, and Claire Kamp Dush. "Fathers' Involvement in Child Health Care: Associations with Prenatal Involvement, Parents' Beliefs, and Maternal Gatekeeping." *Family Relations* 62 (2013): 649–661.

INDEX

ADA. *See* Americans with Disabilities Act

addiction. *See* drug abuse

ADHD, 136, 138, 160–161, 183

Adonis (father), 156–157, 173–174

advertising: for alcohol, 206; for cigarettes, 103–104; for junk food, 99–100, 206

advocacy for child, father's role in: for children with disabilities, 142, 144; with health care professionals, 10, 12, 25, 58, 142, 144, 147–152, 156–157; and helmet safety, 188–189; Internet and, 147–148; need for improvement in, 189; as part of proactive stance, 204

advocacy for mother-to-be, father's role in, 54–55

Affordable Care Act, 205

Agency for Healthcare Research and Quality (AHRQ), 14

aging, men's struggle to accept, 115–116

alcohol: abuse in returned military personnel, 112–113; advertising for, 206; health effects of, 1, 2; and poor parenting, 32

American Academy of Pediatrics, 136, 170, 171

American College of Sports Medicine (ACSM), 93, 94

American Fitness Index (ACSM), 93, 94

Americans with Disabilities Act (ADA), 135–136

America's Most Wanted (TV series), 86

Angelman syndrome, 153–154

Arnie (pediatric pulmonologist), 144–145, 147, 148

Ashkenazi Jews, foodways of, 73

Austin (father), 101–102

autism, children with, 137–138, 154–155, 166; coparenting of, 183; diagnosis of, 138; higher prevalence in males, 136; recent

increase in, 136; training for fathers of, 200–201

Baby Boot Camp, 196

Baby Bump (phone app), 48

Bailey (stay-at-home father), 177–179

Barry (father), 48

Beatie, Thomas, 45

birth experience in hospitals, 54–55

blindness. *See* vision loss/impairment

Blueprint for Men's Health (MHN), 16

bond(s): coaching of youth sports and, 27, 78–79, 203; definition and types of, 22–23; disabilities and, 140, 152–154; exercise with child and, 59; family rituals and, 58, 62; gardening and, 63–65; illness and, 35–36; play in nature and, 30. *See also* father-child partnership

The Boys Initiative, 191–192

breast-feeding: coparenting approach to, 178–179; demographics of, 53–54; fathers' support for, 51, 52, 57; and gender equality, 52–54; need for public health campaigns on, 53; outreach to fathers about, 196–197; research on parents' views, 51–52; vegetarians/vegans and, 216n1

Brent (middle-aged father), 63–64, 66, 75

Brown, Beckie, 189

Bruce (pediatrician), 147

Cadel (Jamaican-Chinese father), 69, 71

Cal (father), 115–116

Campbell (blind father), 117–119, 136, 146–147, 155

car accidents, 84, 89

caregiving by fathers. *See* involvement of father with children

Centers for Disease Control, 103
Chad (father), 107, 143–144, 179
challenges faced by fathers, strategies for
    overcoming, 28. *See also* coparenting;
    financial constraints; illness or injury in
    fathers
Chao (Asian father), 92
Chicagoland (CNN series), 92
childhood influences: and father's view of
    health, 33–38; as importance but not
    definitive, 38–39
children's health: fathers' role in health
    matrix and, 10, 190, 207, 208; impact of
    fathers' health practices on, 8; linking
    fathers' health to, 16–17, 211n32; need
    for programs encouraging in boys, 39;
    obesity increases, 17; poor quality of in
    United States, 4–5; programs to support
    father's role in, 203, 204. *See also* disabili-
    ties; exercise; health care professionals;
    illness of children; injury or death of
    children; proactive involvement of men
    in child's health; *other specific topics*
Children's Trust, 198
chronic complex conditions (CCC), 140,
    147
chronic illness in children, prevalence of, 5.
    See also entries under disabilities
cities: and fitness of poorer families, 195;
    options for fitness activities in, 93
Clive (marathon runner), 109
coaching of youth sports: author and, 3,
    11, 26, 27, 78, 79, 177; and bonding with
    child, 27, 78–79, 203; impact on child's
    success, 79; and models of masculinity,
    78–79
Coakley, Jay, 77–78
Coleman, William, 170
communities, role in good fathering, 202,
    207
community organizations: father as child's
    advocate with, 142; fathers' partnership
    with, 8, 9, 101–102; interventions by, as
    opportunity, 9; programs supporting
    father's role in child's health, 203, 204;
    promotion of health and fitness by, 16;
    support of fitness for poorer families, 195

concussion(s): of author's son, 187–188;
    need for prevention activism, 188–189;
    new awareness of, 13–14, 121, 189
controversial topics, new openness about,
    120–121
Cooper, Anderson, 45
coparenting: breast-feeding and, 178–179;
    of children with disabilities, 24, 160–161,
    179–180, 183; components of, 159; and
    decisions, 175–178; definitions of,
    158–159; extended family and, 163; father
    as child's advocate in, 142; father's role
    in, factors affecting, 163–166; financial
    constraints and, 171–172; gay parents
    and, 159–163; health and fitness and,
    180–186; health care professionals and,
    169–171; increased family fluidity and,
    22; by non-cohabiting parents, issues
    in, 158–163, 167–169, 174; parents' dif-
    ferent strengths and, 182–183; parents'
    relationship and, 8–9, 166–167, 173–174;
    parents' schedules and, 184–185; social
    landscape as context for, 163; technology
    use by child as issue in, 174–175; types of
    interactions in, 163; women health pro-
    fessionals and, 172–173
cultural expectations: impact on men's
    self-conceptions, 26; and men's health,
    18–19
cystic fibrosis, 144–145

Dads & Kids: Health & Fitness Talk (web-
    site), 16–17, 204
Dad to Dad (Hill), 199
Darling-Fisher, Cynthia, 200
Delmore (father), 50
Deutsch, Jonathan, 73
diabetes, 17, 117, 136
Dialogue on Men's Health Conference
    (2012), 16
Diego (father), 50–51
diet and nutrition: in doctors, 125; ethnic
    cuisines, 71–74, 99; family support
    in, 119–120; Fooducate app and, 69,
    122; immigrants' adoption of US diet,
    73, 74; non-cohabiting parents and,
    169; parental conflict about, 183–184;

health care costs, rise in, 206

health care professionals: and coparenting, 169–171, 180–181; father as child's advocate with, 10, 12, 25, 58, 142, 144, 147–152, 156–157; father as mother-to-be's advocate with, 54–55; and father's health, 195–199; on fathers' level of involvement, 10, 144–145, 156; fathers of special needs children and, 24; health and nutrition practices of, 126; and inclusion of fathers, 199–200; interviewed for this study, 10; time constraints on discussing fathers' role, 197, 200; women as, 172–173. *See also* doctors; pediatricians

health-conscious fathers: basic functions of, 58; as proactive, 58, 77; strategies to promote, 201–205. *See also* procreative consciousness; *entries under* proactive

health information: Internet and, 121–122, 147–148, 175, 193–194; parent-child discussions and, 120–121

health matrix: of author's family, 12; benefits of fathers' understanding of, 190; of children, fathers' role in, 10, 190, 207, 208; of coparents, 163, 186; and creation of nurturing fathers, 202; definition of, 5–6; elements of beyond family, 186; factors shaping conception of, 8, 28, 33–39; genetic risk factors and, 122; modification of, to make fathers more welcome, 199–200; reciprocal nature of, 178; socioeconomic context of, 18

Healthy Dads, Healthy Kids program (Australia), 211n32

Healthy Families Massachusetts program, 198

healthy lifestyle, adoption of: children's support for, 204; family as motive for, 39, 42, 118, 120, 124, 127, 128; including child in planning of, 23; in response to child's pressure, 42

helmets, 89–90, 187–189

Hendricks, Justin, 188

Hill, David, 199

hospitals: birth experience in, 54–55; and fathers as advocate for child in, 148–152

Huggies diapers commercial, 164

Hunter (stay-at-home dad), 153–154, 165, 180

The Hunt with John Walsh (TV series), 86

illness of children: coparenting in, 169; father-child partnership in, 35–36, 133; and parental safety concerns, 92. *See also entries under* disabilities

illness or injury in fathers: chronic, lack of support in, 25; as constraint on physical activity, 26–28, 101; isolated problems, 25–26; men's tendency to avoid addressing, 114; range of problems, 25; sense of control over health and, 116–118

injuries, minor, level of reaction to as coparenting decision, 176–178

injury or death of children: causes of, 83, 84–86; emergency room visits per year, 83; fathers' reports of, 82–83, 86–87; media incitement of fears about, 83, 85; risk of, 82

institutional racism, and health, 18

institutions: effects on children with disabilities, 137; influence on definition of health, 7; need to include men in child health matrices, 190; partnerships with as key component in health matrix, 39. *See also* community organizations; government programs

Internet: and child's ability to challenge father, 23–24; percentage of children using, 175; as source of health information, 121–122, 147–148, 175, 193–194

involvement of father with children: changing concept of family and, 20–24; changing gender expectations and, 19–21, 68, 70, 73, 74, 163–164, 201–202, 208; in fathers of children with disabilities, 5, 137, 144–147, 156; health care professionals on level of, 10, 144–145, 156; increase in, 21; modern expectations for, 20; mothers as gatekeepers of, 165; need to encourage, 10; value of, 203. *See also* prenatal period, fathers' involvement in; *entries under* proactive involvement

Jackson (vegan store clerk), 67–68

Jake (father), 138–139, 140, 142–143, 155

ABOUT THE AUTHOR

WILLIAM MARSIGLIO, Ph.D., is a professor in the Department of Sociology and Criminology & Law, University of Florida, and a fellow in the National Council on Family Relations. A leading scholar in the fields of family and fatherhood, he uses a social psychological and gendered perspective to study how men express their identities as fathers and youth workers in various settings. He is the author of more than sixty-five articles and book chapters as well as ten books, including *Nurturing Dads: Social Initiatives for Contemporary Fatherhood* (2012), *Men on a Mission: Valuing Youth Work in Our Communities* (2008), and a novel, *The Male Clock: A Futuristic Novel about a Fertility Crisis, Gender Politics, and Identity* (2015). Marsiglio developed the website *Dads & Kids: Health & Fitness Talk* (http://www .dadsandkidshealth.com/) to promote healthy lifestyles for fathers and children while targeting dads (and moms), youth, teachers, and pediatric health care professionals.